ADHD FAQ

Andrew Coltrin

I0805893

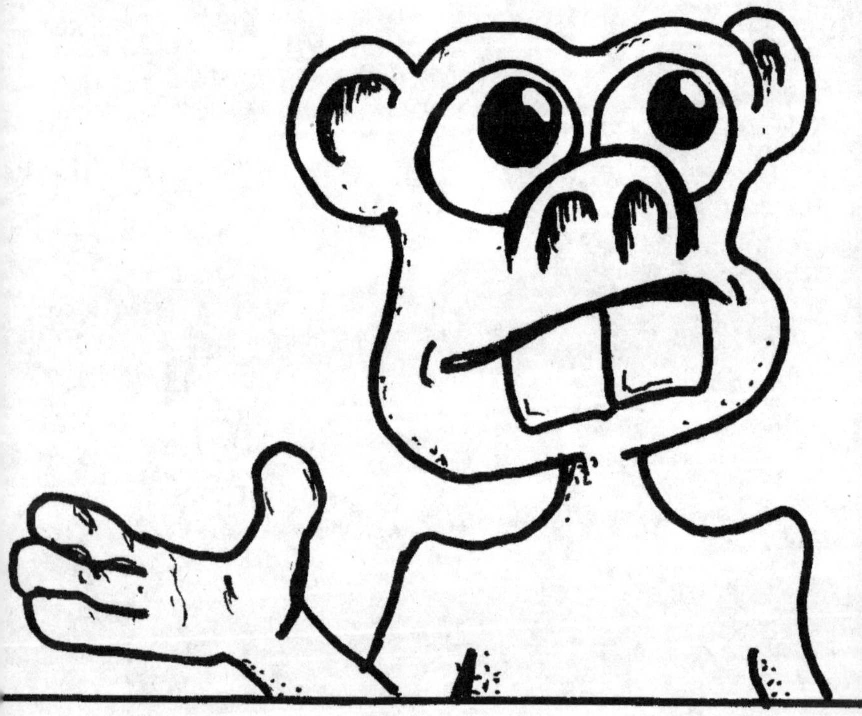

ADHD FAQ

Understand and Embrace Your Brain, from Diagnosis to Everyday Life

Andrew Coltrin
with Dr. Faith G. Harper

Microcosm Publishing
Portland, Oregon | Cleveland, Ohio

ADHD FAQ

Understand and Embrace Your Brain, from Diagnosis to Everyday Life
© Andrew Coltrin, 2026

Foreword © Dr. Faith G. Harper

This edition © Microcosm Publishing 2026
Paperback ISBN 9781648415388

Ebook ISBN 9781648417368

This is Microcosm # 998

Edited by Ivy Zeller

Designed by Joe Biel and Sarah Koch

Illustrated by Andrew Coltrin

For a catalog, write or visit:

Microcosm Publishing

2752 N Williams Ave.

Portland, OR 97227

All the news from the misfits in print at Microcosm.Pub / Newsletter

Get more copies of this book at Microcosm.Pub / ADHDFAQ

EU Safety Information: microcosmpublishing.com / gpsr

To join the ranks of high-class stores that feature Microcosm titles, talk to your rep: In the U.S. COMO (Atlantic), ABRAHAM (Midwest), sales@microcosm.pub (Texas, Oklahoma, Louisiana, Arkansas), IMPRINT (Pacific), TURNAROUND (UK, Africa, Europe, Middle East), UTP / MANDA (Canada), NEWSOUTH (Australia / New Zealand), Sendpoints (Asia), HarperCollins (India), and FAIRE in the gift trade.

Did you know that you can buy our books directly from us at sliding scale rates? Support a small, independent publisher and pay less than Amazon's price at Microcosm.Pub.

Global labor conditions are bad, and our roots in industrial Cleveland in the '70s and '80s made us appreciate the need to treat workers right. Therefore, our books are MADE IN THE USA.

Microcosm's workers and authors are paid solely from book sales. If you downloaded this book from some sketchy part of the internet or picked up what appears to be a bootleg, please support our hardworking team by purchasing a copy directly from us and encouraging your communities to do the same. Paying for our books and zines helps us publish work that's far better than anything AI can come up with. Additionally, a 2025 MIT study revealed that AI inhibits humanity's critical thinking ability. Since critical thinking is one of our core values, we prohibit any use of our books to "train" generative artificial "intelligence" (AI) technologies, because seriously, WTF?

Library of Congress Cataloging-in-Publication Data

Names: Coltrin, Andrew author | Harper, Faith G. writer of foreword

Title: The ADHD FAQ : understand and embrace your brain, from diagnosis to everyday life / by Andrew Coltrin ; foreword by Faith G. Harper.

Other titles: Attention-deficit hyperactivity disorder frequently asked questions

Description: [Portland] : Microcosm Publishing, [2026] | Includes bibliographical references. | Summary: "Everything you ever wanted to ask about ADHD, but kept forgetting to"-- Provided by publisher.

Identifiers: LCCN 2026018624 | ISBN 9781648415388 trade paperback

Subjects: LCSH: Attention-deficit hyperactivity disorder | Attention-deficit hyperactivity disorder in adults

Classification: LCC RC394.A85 C64 2026

LC record available at https://lccn.loc.gov/2026018624"

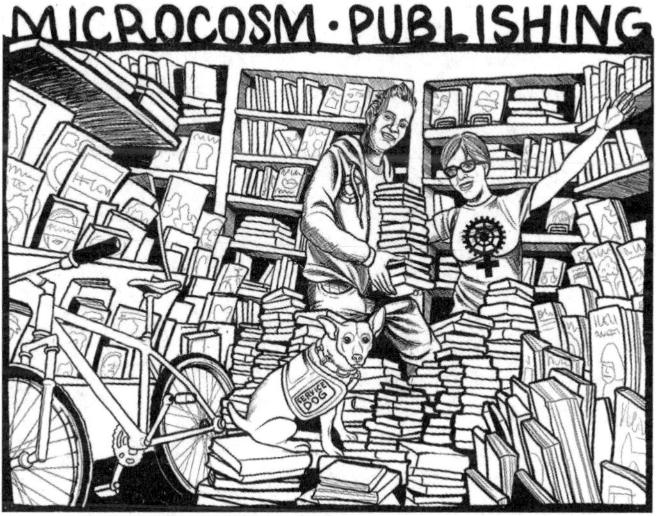

Microcosm Publishing is Portland's most diversified publishing house and distributor, with a focus on the colorful, authentic, and empowering. Our books and zines have put your power in your hands since 1996, equipping readers to make positive changes in their lives and in the world around them. Microcosm emphasizes skill-building, showing hidden histories, and fostering creativity through challenging conventional publishing wisdom with books and bookettes about DIY skills, food, bicycling, gender, self-care, and social justice. What was once a distro and record label started by Joe Biel in a drafty bedroom was determined to be *Publishers Weekly*'s fastest-growing publisher of 2022 and #3 in 2023 and 2024, and is now among the oldest independent publishing houses in Portland, OR, and Cleveland, OH. We are a politically moderate, centrist publisher in a world that has inched to the right for the past 80 years.

FOREWORD BY FAITH G. HARPER

This is a book that Microcosm readers (who are, clearly, the best readers in the world) have been demanding for a hot minute. (This is why y'all are the best readers: you're not the least bit afraid to tell us what's up.) And I got the easiest task of everyone involved . . . I just have to say nice things about the project before you get to the nice things themselves.

Andrew is that great combination of professional experience (he would say paraprofessional since his work has been as an instructional assistant, not a certified teacher), advocacy work, and lived experience. Which is all to say, you are in really good hands here. He knows what the struggles feel like coming from the inside and what the obstacles look like coming from the outside. And let's pasture right there . . . I wanna talk about that for a minute.

Society isn't built for neurodivergent brains to thrive within. Which leads to every neurodivergent person I have ever met feeling like they are failing at life more often than not. And here is the Auntie Faith perspective on that problem. You aren't failing at being a member of society—society has failed and continues to fail at creating a you-shaped space to grow and thrive. Because if being ADHD was such a terrible thing, evolution would have pruned off that particular brain-wiring eleventy-thousand years ago.

There will continue to be problems in the world that can only be solved by a neurodivergent operating system. We don't just want you to stick around, we need you . . . all of us. You're not slowing the neurotypicals down; we've been slowing you down. And it's shitty and it sucks and I'm sorry.

And *that* is where Andrew's book and his variety of perspectives on neurodiversity come in. He's dealt with those same struggles in his own life, and in the lives of kiddos he has worked with and family members he loves. So he's very aware of what options are available, barriers to access, and the emotional fallout of the whole process. And honestly? I can't think of any better writer-advocate to help you understand your experiences based on the best and newest research we have so you can make choices that suit you best. Formal diagnosis or nah? School or work accommodations? Supplements, meds, rawdogging reality?

Many books are going to give you a specific plan about how they think you should handle being ADHD. Andrew is gonna tell you, over and over, that he isn't the boss of you so here's as many options as he can think of so you can make a plan that is tailored to your specific needs. Cuz it isn't like society has your six on that one, right?

Or maybe you are wanting to better understand and support a loved one through their journey. Because you also recognize that we don't have a social structure that is going to ensure those needs are met. (We both love you so much for that, by the way.)

So updated research, options and how to access them, and no stupid influencer bullshit trying to sell you a damn thing. Cuz all we want is for you to have as fulfilling and joyful a life as you can wring out of this world.

So grab your three beverages (one for energy, one for hydration, and one for taste . . . if you're ADHD, you know) and let's get to it!

CONTENTS

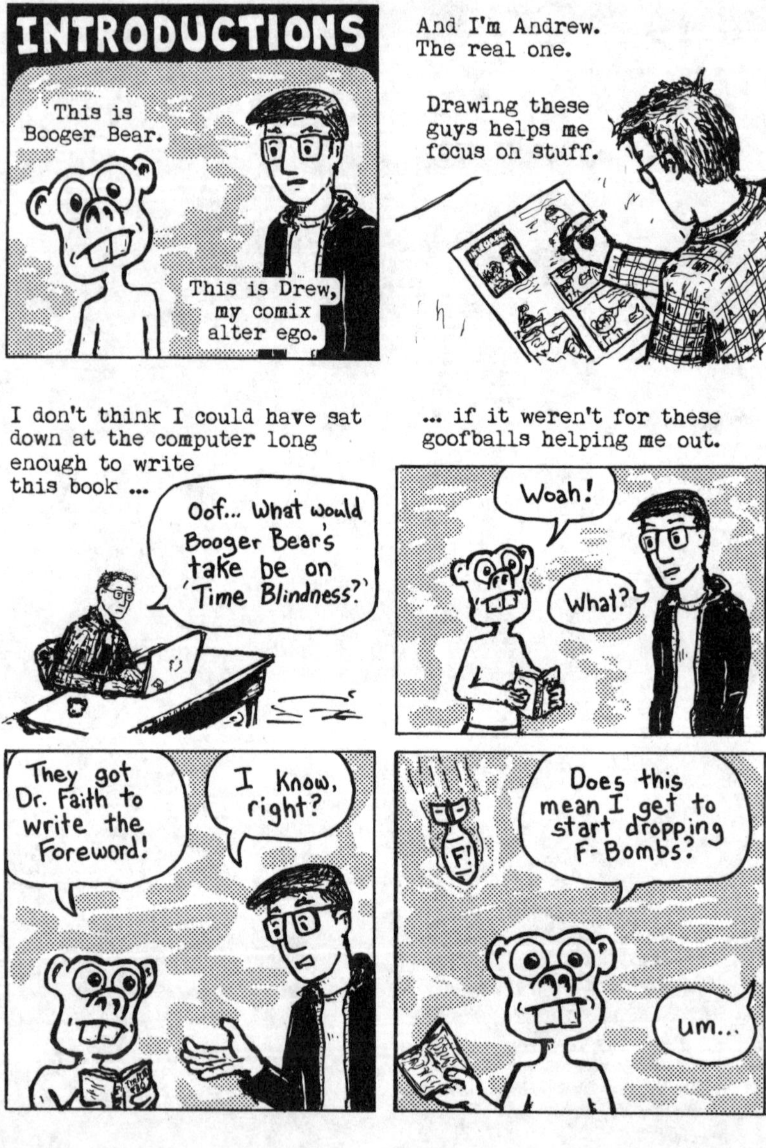
INTRODUCTIONS
This is Booger Bear.
This is Drew, my comix alter ego.
And I'm Andrew. The real one.
Drawing these guys helps me focus on stuff.
I don't think I could have sat down at the computer long enough to write this book ...
Oof... What would Booger Bear's take be on 'Time Blindness?'
... if it weren't for these goofballs helping me out.
Woah!
What?
They got Dr. Faith to write the Foreword!
I Know, right?
F!
Does this mean I get to start dropping F-Bombs?
um...

INTRODUCTION: QUESTIONS RELATED TO THIS BOOK

Have you ever been diagnosed with ADHD?

Is this a question you have for this author, dear reader?

Or is it a question someone has asked you, and you never followed up on it?

Or you did follow up on it, only to find yourself getting some murky doctor-speak information, a stack of unread articles, and another stack of unused day planners—and even after all that, still struggling with the same struggles you've always struggled with?

Or maybe it's a question you have about someone in your life.

Which all leads to the scary-ish question within the question, "Should I ask a professional if I have ADHD?"

In all of these cases, I'm glad you found this book. You are who I wrote it for.

I also wrote it for myself, because I've had all these same questions as a fellow ADHDer.

As a Neurodiversity advocate, I believe that ADHD is one of the many threads in the diverse tapestry of human existence. ADHD is part of who we *Homo sapiens* are as a whole, but it's a part that has been hidden away and disguised with euphemisms, social masking, and a strange compulsion to hide any diversions from the neurotypical strands in the tapestry. And, history has shown, whenever humans try to hide a difference in themselves or others, there's a lot of unnecessary suffering that occurs.

It's amazing how much suffering a person will put up with if they have no idea that the majority of others do not suffer in the same way.

Like most of my writing, my goal with this book is to increase understanding and to reduce suffering.

What makes me qualified to write this book?

Short answer: hands-on life experience coupled with insatiable curiosity.

Long answer: I've been writing about neurodivergence and been an advocate for the Neurodiversity Movement ever since I confirmed my autistic nature back in 2012. At that moment in clinical psychology history, it was the prevailing practice that a person could be either autistic or ADHD, but not both. So, the fact that I was, at that time, highly motivated to get an autism diagnosis effectively turned my attention away from my ADHD traits.

But life experience kept bringing me into contact with ADHDers.

As the Neurodiversity Movement grew, and more ADHDers found a place among the autistics who started it, we found we had a lot in common and a lot we could learn from each other. One autistic friend of mine pointed out that she's observed a trend where autistic people often have a close friend who has ADHD.

In my work as a special education paraeducator, I've observed this phenomenon on the playground. With a decade and a half of working with students with a variety of disabilities, I've picked up some practical knowledge on what ADHD looks like from the outside, sussed out how it's affecting students on the inside, and provided the right nudges and supports to help those students stay on track in the very challenging sensory environment of the typical classroom.

In the last couple years, my Neurodiversity social media feeds started bringing me more stories from people diagnosed with both autism and ADHD, which opened my eyes to the fact that it was a possibility to be AuDHD. Of course, memes and hashtags are far from official qualifications. When I started having extra trouble at work after a welcome addition to my family turned all my home routines upside down, I talked to some behavioral health professionals and my primary care physician. So, I got to confirm that, in addition to being autistic, I've been struggling to manage ADHD on my own and in the dark for almost fifty years. That's got to count for something.

Who is this book for?

I want to make sure you know this book is for you. Big picture, this book is for anyone who is curious about ADHD. Of course, everyone's curiosity is going to come from a different place.

I know some readers will be looking at this book because they are curious if they themselves might have ADHD. Been there. Done that. I got you.

Some readers will look to this book for answers to questions they have about family members who have been diagnosed. Sometimes those family members will be children. Parents have a lot of questions. I know. I'm a parent. And I have a child with ADHD. I got you.

I also have some firsthand insight into how the school system works, and doesn't work, for kids with ADHD. Oh boy, buckle up.

And, adults with or without a formal diagnosis? Who want some tips on how to manage the things that come up in life? This book is for you too.

Let's go on a curiosity journey together.

How do I read this book?

I did not write this book straight through from beginning to end. I don't expect anyone to read it straight through, but you can. That's fine.

Questions and answers are arranged into sections according to which domain of life they relate to. Sometimes an answer will refer to a question in a different section of the book. It's totally okay to jump around from section to section, letting your curiosity be your guide. If there's a bit that doesn't apply to you or doesn't interest you, I'm not offended if you want to skip it.

That being said, my goal is to write from a lived-experience perspective, in plain language, in a way that is accessible to as many people as possible. I will do my best to explain the complicated and science-heavy medical terms as they come up. I'll also illuminate the hashtags and Neurodiversity insider terms that will undoubtedly pepper my writing.

ADHD 101

In this section, we'll cover the basics about the world of ADHD, from language choices to statistics about how prevalent ADHD is to debunking some common misconceptions, and more!

What terms should we use when we talk about people with ADHD?

There are a few schools of thought on this one.

The first one states that "person-first" language needs to be used at all times and in all circumstances. Person-first language follows the example of saying "a person with a disability" rather than "a disabled person." This is usually considered best practice among professionals with licenses regulated by government entities. There are also a lot of parents who want to make sure their child is seen as a whole person outside of the disability. Some of these parents like to hire lawyers to sue government entities, like public school districts, when they don't treat their children fairly. So, the person-first language gets adopted as the professional standard because it's one more layer of interference to keep the parents with the lawyers at bay. (This last little factoid is from my inside experience of working in public schools for fifteen years. There is a hyper-awareness on the part of special education teachers and school-based case managers regarding the litigious nature of some parents.)

Then there is the "identity-first" language school of thought. This school of thought is rooted in the blind and deaf communities. When person-first language started becoming best professional practice, many blind people and deaf people rejected it, because calling themselves people with visual impairments and people with hearing impairments really belittled what they felt was a core part of their identities. Being blind or deaf, they argued, was as formative to who they are as what culture they are born into. They identify as blind and deaf, so it makes no sense for them to be labeled differently. This line of thinking was quickly adopted by the autistic community as soon as they found each other on the internet and realized there was an autistic community. Also, a lot of autistic people felt like saying "person who has autism" is not only grammatically awkward (passive voice), but it's inefficient, using three or four words when one or two do the job just fine.

Which school is right? It depends on the context and who you are talking to.

In both these schools, you can see where the function of the terminology lies. Person-first language tends to originate from outside the people it is talking about, while the identity-first language tends to be preferred by the people themselves.

In the case of ADHD, the term is more grammatically problematic than blind, deaf, or autistic. It's an initialism, rather than a proper word in its own right. It almost insists on being used in the person-first formation because it isn't obvious how to make an adjective out of it. However, English speakers have never backed down from an opportunity to coin a neologism. Thus we have the word ADHDer, meaning a person who is ADHD. Also, if you notice, I wrote *is* instead of *has.* Me saying "I am ADHD" is the identity-first way to get away from that dreaded passive voice problem.

Some ADHDers have a very strong preference for saying *am* as opposed to *have.*

In my writing, I will shift constantly between all these language choices, largely due to the context of the passage at hand. In real life, I like to respect the language preferences of the specific person I'm talking to or about. But, also, in real life, sometimes I'm just glad the words come out of my mouth in an understandable order.

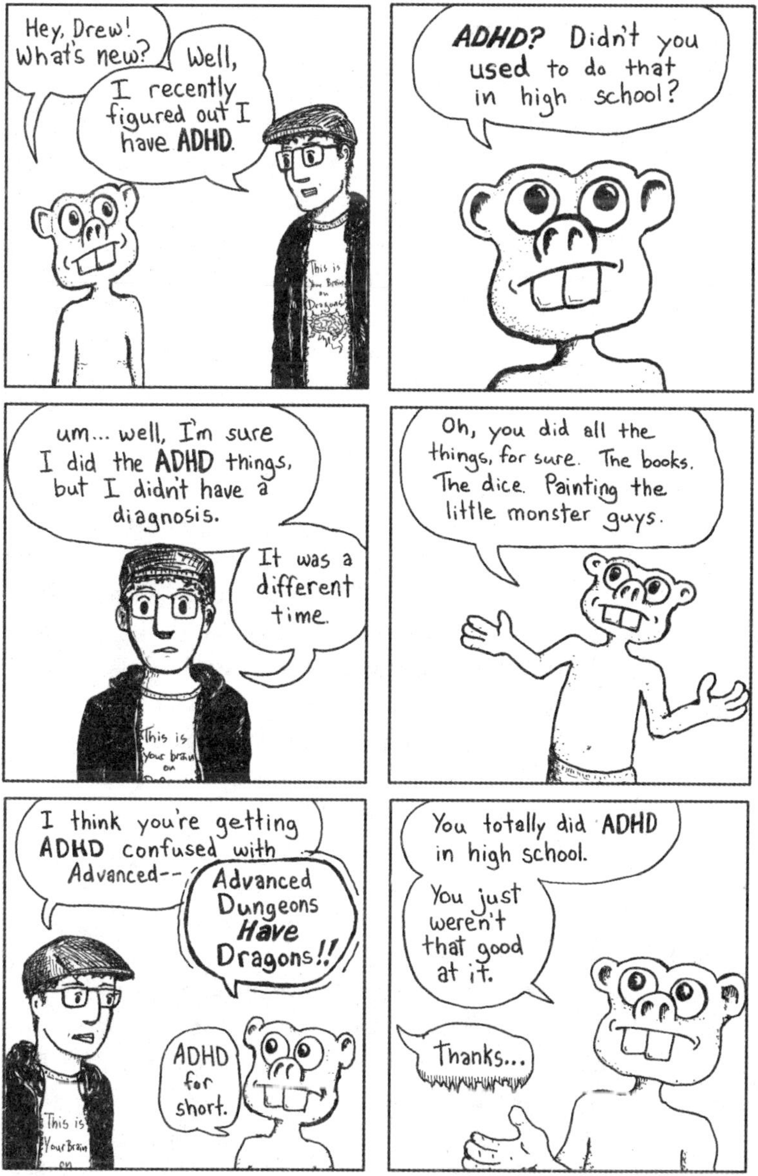
Hey, Drew! What's new?
Well, I recently figured out I have ADHD.
ADHD? Didn't you used to do that in high school?
um... well, I'm sure I did the ADHD things, but I didn't have a diagnosis.
It was a different time.
Oh, you did all the things, for sure. The books. The dice. Painting the little monster guys.
I think you're getting ADHD confused with Advanced--
Advanced Dungeons Have Dragons!!
ADHD for short.
You totally did ADHD in high school.
You just weren't that good at it.
Thanks...

How common is ADHD?

ADHD is about as common as left-handedness. About 1 in every 10 people (10%) is left-handed, and this percentage has been consistent in times and places where left-handedness is not stigmatized. The CDC reports, based on a recent study of data gathered in 2022, that 11.4% of children in the United States have had an ADHD diagnosis.[1] So, if you know enough people to know some lefties, you know enough people to have someone with ADHD in your circle.

(At the time of this writing, there's a lot of confusion going on at the CDC. I can't have confidence that pages on the CDC website that had good information in 2024 still have good information in 2026.)

What does ADHD stand for?

That initialism is short for "Attention-Deficit/Hyperactivity Disorder." This is a collection of medical diagnostic terms that are both misleading and kind of derogatory. These terms reflect a decades-old bias in medicine and psychology that there is a baseline standard of normal for human beings and we all should endeavor to approach that baseline of normalcy. If you take a look at the individual words, they definitely imply that someone with ADHD is missing something (deficit) and that something's wrong with how they do things (disorder). Pretty rude.

There is also a lot of confusion about how the terms poorly reflect the lived experience of ADHDers. I'd been hearing about ADHD for a long time, but had trouble seeing it as something that reflected me, because I don't have a deficit of attention. I'm paying attention to everything. All the time. Sometimes I'm paying attention to something so hard I forget to eat lunch. And as for hyperactivity? No one I know would describe me as hyperactive. Sure, my brain might be on fire sometimes (while my body is reclined and statue-

1 "Data and Statistics on ADHD," Attention-Deficit/Hyperactivity Disorder (ADHD), November 19, 2024, https://www.cdc.gov/adhd/data/index.html.

still on the couch), but I'm hardly ever jumping out of my seat and climbing the walls.

What does ADHD do to you?

I'm going to have to unpack this question a bit because, first of all, ADHD isn't something that happens to people, it's a part of how some people are built. So, in one sense, ADHD isn't doing anything to an ADHDer.

However, the traits of an ADHDer are very difficult to incorporate into the everyday life of late-stage capitalism in a western market economy. Except for when those ADHD traits are assets. Which sometimes they are. So, this question is now begetting other questions, and I haven't even broken down the first question yet.

So, basically, ADHD isn't something that happens to you, it's something you are. Depending on a multitude of factors—like the strategies you've learned from your family of origin, the strategies you've intuitively created for yourself, your cultural background, your economic status, and any other neurodivergent or medical conditions you might have—the traits of ADHD can express themselves in so many ways, it can be difficult to identify and address.

So, a better question would be . . .

What are the flavors of ADHD?

Okay. I made this question up, because I didn't want to use the words *symptom, trait,* or *presentation.* Every time I tried to answer questions with those words, my own inner gremlins objected. *Flavor* is a word the gremlins aren't having a problem with.

Wait a minute. What do you mean by "gremlins"?

Sorry for forcing a subquestion. I'm speaking metaphorically. I don't actually have gremlins inside me. But, I do like peppering my daily life with folkloric concepts.

The concept of the gremlin popped into existence in the early twentieth century among RAF pilots. Airplanes are complicated machines that operate in difficult conditions in order to defy gravity. Parts break, accidents happen, and it sure is nice to blame a nonhuman imp that likes to sabotage airplanes rather than channel your anger at the other human members of your team. Humans generally don't like having anger channeled at them. Folkloric concepts are a bit more resilient.

So, when my brain gets stuck, and I'm having too much trouble moving forward in a direction that, objectively, shouldn't be that difficult? Obviously, my inner gremlins have been cutting wires and doing other acts of sabotage that affect my brain's workings.

My workaround is to try and find a new, clever, or exciting twist to get myself back into a productive groove. In this case, I came up with the idea of ADHD having flavors.

Can you get back to the flavors of ADHD, please?

Of course. According to the big fat book of clinical terms, the DSM-5, ADHD has three main presentations (flavors): inattentive, hyperactive/impulsive, and combined. Of these terms, *combined* is both the least insulting and the most confusing. I'm not a big fan of insulting and confusing terminology, but these are the industry standards, so let's stick with them for now.

The predominantly inattentive type is what used to be called ADD. The traits according to the big, fat industry manual include: failing to give close attention to details or making careless mistakes, trouble paying attention, not seeming to listen when spoken to directly, not following through on instructions and failing to finish tasks, having trouble organizing tasks or activities, avoiding tasks that require sustained attention, losing things, being easily distracted, and being forgetful in daily activities.

The predominantly hyperactive/impulsive type is what puts the *H* in ADHD. (It used to be referred to as "hyperkinetic reaction of childhood.") The traits, according to the big, fat book, are fidgeting or squirming, not staying seated when it's keep-your-butt-in-the-chair time, running around or climbing things at inappropriate times, being unable to participate in leisure activities quietly, being often "on-the-go," talking excessively, blurting, trouble waiting one's turn, and interrupting and intruding on others often.

Then there's the combined type. This basically means the ADHDer has enough traits from both the inattentive list and the hyperactive/impulsive list to be considered combined.

I've paraphrased the big, fat book because it's kind of boring, repetitive, and, in my opinion, judgy. The DSM is focused on how ADHD is perceived from the outside and is designed to help clinicians make accurate diagnostic judgements. So, it's supposed to be judgy.

I'm not a clinician, so I don't have to like it. I prefer perspectives that are informed by the internal experiences of people who have some pretty strong insights into what goes on inside their own heads.

That being said, the big, fat book is a very important reference in determining who would benefit from what kind of treatment. But, even as I was typing up the lists of inattentive and hyperactive/impulsive traits, I couldn't help but ask, "Aren't these just the same things, just some turned inward and some turned outward?"

And the obvious answer is, yes. They are all part of the same thing; that's why the American Psychological Association used years of compiled data and analysis to guide their decision to change their terminology and diagnosis criteria to make this clearer with every revision of the DSM. It's all part of the same thing, but there are different flavors, especially if you look at it from the outside.

What are the common ADHD traits in everyday language?

I've put off answering this one because it's kind of hard on my self-esteem. But, here goes. First, the negative stuff: poor executive function (trouble making decisions and getting started on stuff), poor self-regulation, overloaded working memory, time-blindness, trouble finishing tasks, overcommitting yourself, underperforming, staying up too late, drinking lots of coffee, craving input, absolutely dreading boredom, trouble sitting still, having body aches,and experiencing irritability. As an adult, the big symptom that manifests in ADHDers who haven't been diagnosed yet is unexplained underachievement.

Unexplained underachievement is the thing where someone who was in the gifted program at school as a child winds up dropping out of college, bounces around between retail and service industry jobs, talks about trying out for *Jeopardy* but always misses the application window, and can't really pinpoint the exact moment where everything went wrong. There is also often some sort of substance abuse problem thrown into this mix. This is not the destiny of every undiagnosed ADHDer, but it does happen a lot. In my own case, I worked at coffee shops and used bookstores for a long time before finding my way into working a public education job in my thirties.

And, of course, demure, semi-ace, autistic me pussyfooted around a big one that Dr. Faith reminded me to clarify: "Out of control sexual behavior is also common in unmanaged ADHD. Sexologists always screen for ADHD if being a ho-dawg is the chief complaint."

And now that my writerly self-esteem needs a pick-me-up, let's run down some of the positive ADHD traits: high energy, strong will, creativity and imagination, generosity, creepily accurate intuitive leaps, and a quirky sense of humor.

The traits of ADHD often fall into the "it's a gift and a curse" duality. There are some really strong, amazing qualities that let ADHDers excel in areas that are difficult for neurotypicals to match. But those are counterbalanced by the impulsiveness and organizational problems that lead us to quit jobs and relationships or get fired more often than neurotypicals.

We have a sense of our amazingness, but we also have front-row seats to our shortcomings, which leads to a lot of negative self-image problems. The disconnect between our mode of being extremely insightful, imaginative, and productive—and our mode of being disorganized, lost in time, and unpredictable—is profound. It stares us in the face every day. It makes us put off getting started with the day until the very last second because we can't screw anything up if we haven't gotten out of bed yet. And, until we learn how to deal with this disconnect as a function of how our brains work differently than most of the brains around us, we hate ourselves for feeling so broken.

This is as true for children with ADHD as it is with adults. In my day job, I've seen too many kids beating themselves up and writing themselves off as failures before they get to fifth grade. And it's all because their ADHD modes of being don't fit in with the expectations of the neurotypical majority paradigm.

What's going on inside the brain that causes ADHD?

In the simplest terms, some of the mechanisms that direct the signals between different parts of the ADHD brain are super quirky. Some people like to compare the ADHD brain to a sports car with a really powerful engine, but dodgy brakes. But sometimes the ADHD brain can be more like a modern fighter jet that needs ten to twenty hours of maintenance for every hour of flight. (This might actually be a more accurate analogy for the AuDHD brain, which requires consistent application of both autism and ADHD maintenance routines.) When everything's going right, the ADHD brain works really, really well and can accomplish things that other brains struggle with. However, the ADHD brain is also susceptible to crashing and burning suddenly and without warning.

Now, stepping aside from the analogy of high performance vehicles, what exactly is going on in the ADHD brain?

First off, let's talk about two networks within the brain that exist within everybody. The first is the task-positive network, or the TPN. This network includes the parts of the brain that get engaged when a person is getting to work on something. This is what's driving the action when someone gets into a flow state. Doing the job is engaging and possibly even satisfying, even if it isn't necessarily pleasant. The brain is able to stay on track because the task is either rewarding in itself, or it sets the stage for an important external reward. This is the function of the brain that keeps your butt in the chair till the job is done, or until the clock on the wall says it's quitting time. Getting into that TPN flow state can be very efficient and productive if we can stay there.

The TPN is contrasted by a different network, the default mode network or the DMN. The default mode network gets engaged when the brain is doing more imaginative or reflective thinking. This is when we take a moment to consider our relationships with others, our future, our past, what went wrong, what went right, and what we'd like to try the next time we're in a similar situation. It's a very useful network because humans are complicated creatures aware of our pasts and futures and trying to coordinate our efforts within complex and competing social structures. The DMN state is also where creative ideas are hatched. It's what kicks in when a person is daydreaming. It's also what kicks in when a person is obsessing, ruminating, and worrying. I've got a hunch it's also a big player in the modern habit of doom-scrolling.

So, in the standard, neurotypical factory-model-sedan of a brain, the transition between using the TPN and DMN is pretty reliable most of the time. A neurotypical can spend two and a half hours diligently plugging away at the corporate drudgery (TPN), take a fifteen-minute coffee break and let the mind wander (DMN), then come back to their work station and get back into TPN mode without too much trouble. When one network is on, the other one is off. It's not too hard to switch between the modes when the situation calls for it. Neurotypicals have it so easy.

ADHDers, on the other hand, have a quirky neurotransmitter situation. The switches between the TPN and the DMN are super glitchy. The brain has a hard time staying in TPN without popping into DMN at the slightest provocation.

In my daily life, I have trouble staying in TPN every time I pass through a doorway. I may have a very simple task in mind like, "go into the garage and get a screwdriver." I can get to the door to the garage just fine, but when I pass through? The DMN starts revving up trying to engage the memory of what my plan was. "I know I came for a tool, but which one? And while I'm here, why don't I grab the drill? And, what the hell, I've been meaning to re-caulk that crack above the built-in bookshelves. Maybe I should think about touch-up paint while I'm at it. But then I'd have to get on my painting clothes. Nope, better not." *Sets down caulk and caulk gun before going back into the house with the drill in my hand.* And passing through that doorway, suddenly the TPN pops back into gear and, DMNit! I don't have that screwdriver I came in for.

This type of scenario gets even more hilarious when it involves getting something from upstairs and I happen to talk to a family member when I'm up there. I get a lot of steps in during the day.

In the ADHD brain, a lot of the struggles can be explained by this slipping between brain networks. It is so hard to get the brain to cooperate on working on a straightforward task for a couple hours straight. However, if the task at hand involves creativity, or imagination, this tendency to frequently slip between modes can actually be an asset.

But, at the same time, the glitchy switches can work the other way. ADHDers are known to get stuck in one or the other of the networks without being able to easily transition out. The inattentive flavor of ADHD is really an outward presentation of being stuck in the DMN mode. The spaciness and lost-in-a-daydream qualities that are the hallmarks of inattentive type ADHD are happening because the DMN is refusing to disengage. And, on the opposite side of that coin, when an ADHDer gets hyperfocused on a task, to the point that they lose track of time, miss meals, and forget to pick up the kids from school, that's a sure sign that the TPN switch is stuck in the on position. Anything that is not right in front of them and part of the task at hand might as well not exist.

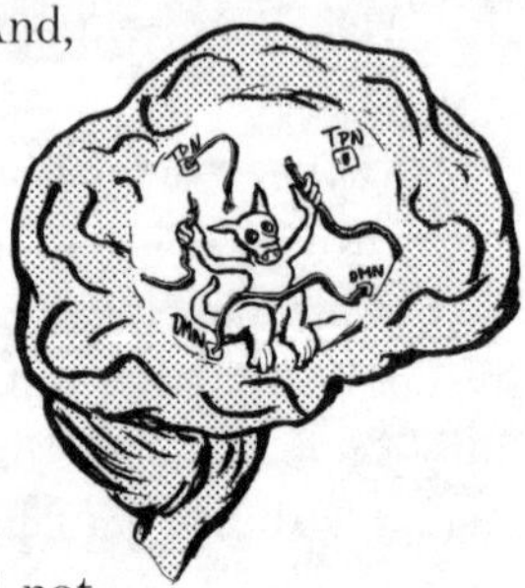

Of course, because ADHD is an extra fun kind of Neurodiversity full of paired dualities and paradoxes, it's not a simple matter of having trouble being in one brain network or the other. Sometimes, in the ADHD brain, both networks are engaged at the same time. Sounds exhausting, right? That's because it is.

Is there a better term for ADHD?

Not yet. Many people agree it's not the best term, but there's no real consensus on what a better term would be.

The term *VAST*[2] (variable attention stimulus trait) has been proposed by Edward Hallowell, MD, and John Ratey, MD—ADHDers, psychiatrists, and authors of *Driven to Distraction* and *ADHD 2.0*. Of course, this term comes with a caveat. In 2022's *ADHD 2.0*, Hallowell and Ratey actually use *VAST* as a term to describe the ever-increasing and noticeable tendencies of neurotypical people to exhibit more ADHD-like traits in our current over-connected, multitasking, screen-facing culture. So, according to Hallowell and Ratey, VAST is different from ADHD, but the traits are similar enough that a lot of the strategies work for both. In a more recent piece in *ADDitude Magazine* (June 2024), they make the case for *VAST* replacing the term

2 Edward Hallowell, MD, "ADHD Needs a Better Name. We Have One.," ADDitude, November 3, 2025, https://www.additudemag.com/attention-deficit-disorder-vast/.

Side Quest: **Cognitive Disengagement Syndrome**

Uh, oh! There's a whole other attention disorder brewing. Dr. Faith tipped me off that Russell Barkley, PhD, is a leading researcher in the effort to discern a distinct kind of attention disorder called Cognitive Disengagement Syndrome (used to be called Sluggish Cognitive Tempo, but they've workshopped it a bit since then). It isn't in the DSM yet, but I don't doubt it's coming. Basically, it has some similarities to the inattentive ADHD presentation (flavor) but it really is proving to be a distinct thing. So, rather than being conveniently explained by the metaphor of having a glitchy switch between TPN and DMN, Cognitive Disengagement Syndrome (CDS) is a more pronounced daydreaminess and lost-in-the-fog way of being, combined with fatigue and being slower to get the body moving. If you are feeling like you only identify with some of the inattention issues of ADHD, but not some of the other stuff, it might be CDS. The bad news is that, since it isn't in the DSM yet, even if your diagnoser knows about CDS, they'll probably put "ADHD, inattentive type" on your paperwork to make the insurance stooges happy.

But don't despair. If your diagnoser is current enough on ADHD information to know about CDS, they can help you find strategies that work for you. The ADHD meds might not work (one big tell that it might actually be CDS and not ADHD), but the loads of non-medication strategies may also be helpful. (I personally think a lot of these strategies can be helpful for anybody.)

Most importantly, you're not alone, and people are working on it. There is a growing body of information out there, and Russell Barkley has some good, lecture-type stuff about it on YouTube.

ADHD altogether.

It's hard to say if *VAST* will take hold. People like to cling to old terms. Case in point: the very magazine in which they are making the case hasn't adjusted its name to reflect the terminology change from *ADD* to *ADHD* that happened in 1987. If *ADHDitude* isn't seen as a viable magazine title, I imagine *VASTitude* probably wouldn't do so well on the newsstands either.

Another interesting term, coming from outside the medical professional arena, is Can't Live Up to Your Bullshit Expectations Syndrome.[3] I like the sentiment, but *CLUYBES* doesn't really roll off the tongue.

And ADHD TikToker Connor DeWolfe made a fun video proposing Dopamine Attention Variability Executive-Dysfunction, or *DAVE*. That sounds fun. Especially because it reminds me of the old Cheech and Chong routine. It would probably be super confusing in real life, which kind of adds to its appeal, if you ask me.

Time will tell if the next inevitable DSM update will give us a new medical term. But will we want to take it up?

Even though Attention-Deficit/Hyperactivity Disorder doubles down on the language of the medical deficit model, I think the letters *ADHD* have some energy to them. I also like that the robot in Dav Pilkey's *Dog Man* books is named 80-HD (a tongue-in-cheek reference to the author's own diagnosis).

There is a precedent for labels of a derogatory origin being reclaimed and reappropriated by the groups they were placed on. The words *queer, punk, nerd, yankee*, and *Methodist* are all examples of pejorative terms that were taken back and turned into positives for the groups they represent.

And also? If they change the term from *ADHD*, I'll have to rewrite this entire book. For the time being, I hope people can appreciate the sentiment that being an ADHDer is pretty punk rock.

---

3 ADDitude Editors, "Does ADHD Need a New Name?", ADDitude, May 9, 2025, https://www.additudemag.com/other-names-for-adhd-add/.

How long does ADHD last?

Short answer, forever. It's a lifelong experience.

It used to be thought that ADHD was something that just affected kids, but they would eventually grow out of it. This line of thinking went hand in hand with the line of thinking that mental health issues are shameful and should never be discussed outside the doors of a therapist's office. These aren't very helpful lines of thinking. ADHD isn't something a person overcomes or endures, it's part of who they are.

Part of the reason it was assumed that ADHD is something people grow out of is that the more visible hyperactivity traits settle down a bit as the prefrontal cortex of the brain finally takes its full adult form around age twenty-five. At this age, human brains in general are a lot better at impulse control. Another factor is that energy levels overall change over the lifespan. The older you get, your metabolism changes, how you spend your energy changes, and the sum of all those little injuries accrued starts slowing you down. All of this contributes to a gradual shift in many ADHDers from the hyperactive-type presentations or combined-type presentations (flavors) to the inattentive-type presentations.

The DSM has been a little quicker to pick up on this new understanding than the ICD (the World Health Organization's diagnostic manual). Which means diagnostic results may vary depending on which manual your diagnoser operates under.

Why are there so many misconceptions about ADHD?

I've got two answers for this one. There are probably loads more, but I'm sticking with two.

First off, ADHD is by its nature full of contradictions. Lots of these contradictions come with a visible aspect and a less visible one. For example, the dreamy space cadet mode of low focus can be pretty obvious from the outside. But, the opposite side of the coin is a preternatural ability to hyperfocus on an urgent project with a hard deadline in twenty-four hours. For every ADHD trait that presents as a potential liability, there's a corresponding trait that can be channeled into functioning as a powerful asset. In the words of TV detective Adrian Monk, "It's a gift . . . and a curse." Unfortunately, for many, the curse is more noticeable than the gift, which leads to misconceptions.

And, now, let me get out my neurodivergent advocacy soapbox so I can properly deliver my second answer:

The prevailing misconceptions about ADHD are so ubiquitous simply because of the sheer number of neurotypical people out there doing the misconceiving. When taking into account all the different neurodivergencies that exist, which is tricky in itself, the rule of thumb is that 15% to 20% of all people are neurodivergent. This means that 80% to 85% of all humans are neurotypical. Neurotypicals tend to operate on the baseline assumption that everyone else they interact with has a brain that works just like theirs. And, because the probability is solidly there, this is a correct assumption on their part at a minimum of 80% of the time. A proper statistician would know how to calculate the variables involved with what sorts of people neurotypicals are likely to interact with and with what regularity. Don't forget to take into account that a certain amount of neurodivergent people would likely not leave their homes or interact with unknown individuals without masking their neurodivergencies super hard. In the hands of someone with more than high school math and some community college accounting classes, that number probably actually approaches something in the 99% range.

So, basically, neurotypicals have an experientially-reinforced confirmation bias toward making the assumption that everybody else's brain works the same.

What are the misconceptions about ADHD?

First up, we have the big, behavioral misconception that ADHDers

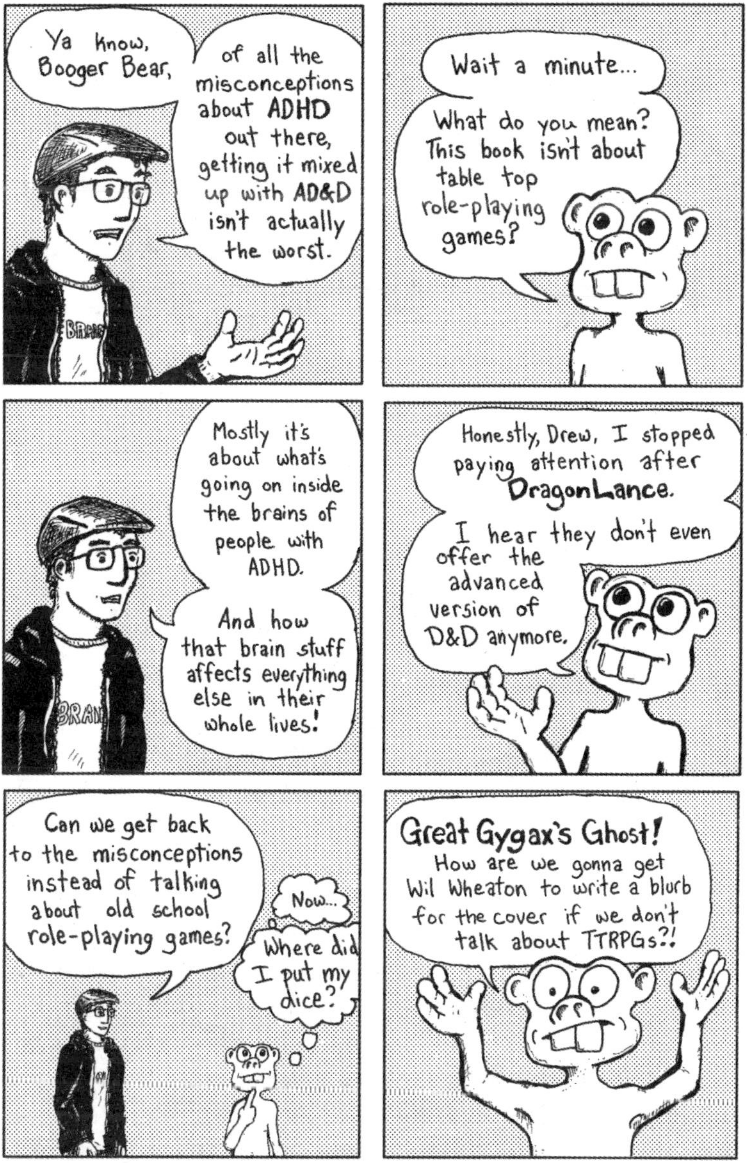
Ya know, Booger Bear,
of all the misconceptions about ADHD out there, getting it mixed up with AD&D isn't actually the worst.
Wait a minute...
What do you mean? This book isn't about table top role-playing games?
Mostly it's about what's going on inside the brains of people with ADHD.
And how that brain stuff affects everything else in their whole lives!
Honestly, Drew, I stopped paying attention after DragonLance.
I hear they don't even offer the advanced version of D&D anymore.
Can we get back to the misconceptions instead of talking about old school role-playing games?
Now...
Where did I put my dice?
Great Gygax's Ghost!
How are we gonna get Wil Wheaton to write a blurb for the cover if we don't talk about TTRPGs?!

are just being lazy and lack the discipline to keep their mouths shut and their butts in their chair. This comes up a lot because I think neurotypicals all really want to be lazy, shout out whatever's on their mind no matter what they might be interrupting, and skip work and run around doing whatever. I think this because I've observed that whenever neurotypicals think they can get away with these things, those things are exactly what they do.

The truth is, your beloved ADHDer will likely get very upset with you if you even suggest they're being lazy about something. The undiagnosed ADHDer is often very self-conscious of the fact that they have to do so much mental work to keep themselves at their current level of productivity. It is literally exhausting, and they tend to feel miserable about disappointing themselves and everyone around them so often. The diagnosed ADHDer will possibly feel similarly but will also have the language to express where you can shove your ableist ideas about what constitutes as lazy.

Next is the misconception where people think ADHD is just a childhood phase that kids grow out of. Sorry. ADHD is pretty much a part of how the ADHDer's brain functions their whole life long. Adults are just better at applying management strategies than kids are. Also, many ADHDers don't get identified as children.

There's also the worry that ADHD meds turn kids into listless zombies. I'm going to draw on my fifteen years experience working in public schools in Arizona and Oregon to say, no. Kids with ADHD are definitely not turning into zombies when they're on their meds. That being said, it is a tricky process to get the dosage right with rapidly changing child bodies and metabolisms. Also, there are a variety of medication options, and figuring out which one works the best for any individual can take time. And there is the issue that stimulant medications can suppress the appetite and there can be a co-occurring slowing of growth for a year or two. So, yes there are things to look out for with the meds, but ideally the parents have a good and productive relationship with the prescribing doctor.

And the flipside of that misconception coin: The ADHD meds solve everything. Nope. Sorry. The meds definitely do some heavy lifting in helping the ADHD brain stay on track, but you still need to do some work to find the tools and supports that allow you to pick which track to be on and when.

Another misconception is that people with ADHD are ideally suited to using their highly activated nervous systems to solve murders as contract consultants to police. This misconception is perpetuated by ADHD-coded characters on popular television shows that wildly exaggerate the amount of murders that go on in an average American city.

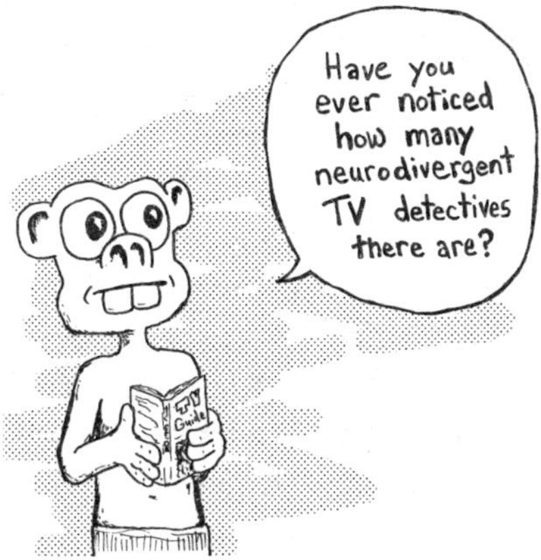
Have you ever noticed how many neurodivergent TV detectives there are?

Of course, the biggest misconception is that ADHD is something that primarily affects boys. This isn't true. Cis boys just happen to get diagnosed in childhood more frequently than cis girls.

Why aren't girls diagnosed with ADHD as frequently as boys?

This phenomenon has its roots in the outdated, but stubbornly entrenched, scientific misunderstanding that, medically, women are pretty much the same as men, only smaller. This is not true. I don't know how or why this ever happened. Because cis female bodies go through profoundly different things than cis male bodies do: menstruation, childbirth, and menopause, to name a few. All of these have ramifications on the same brain chemistry processes that are part of ADHD. It seems stupid to ignore data from half the available sample set, but that's what they did for a long time.

Because the diagnostic criteria was, for so long, focused on how ADHD presents in boys, there really wasn't much effort put into asking how it might present differently in girls. There's a similar phenomenon with autism. The research started out with a pile of gender bias baked in. It's getting better as more data is collected with refined tools and focus. But, as the newest scientific information tends to take decades to filter through the professional community, through tangential professions, and onto the public at large, there are a lot of people walking around with outdated information in their heads. These are often the same people who cling to the most ancient texts for their moral and philosophical instruction.

Could this still be the work of the patriarchy? Not sure, but it definitely works in the patriarchy's favor.

But, who it definitely doesn't work for are the generations of ADHD girls and young women who were misdiagnosed with mood disorders. These girls and women struggled with inappropriate medications, shame, and a twofold sense of failure as human beings. Twofold because (1) they had all the struggles with functioning in the world that ADHD gave them, and (2) they were not seeing any improvement from being treated for a mood disorder.

Taking it another layer further, it's the hyperactive-impulsive and combined flavors of ADHD that are more often identified in childhood. The inattentive flavor can go unnoticed for a long time, because its expression is mostly internal. Now, whether it's a factor of biology or culture, I'm not sure, but historically, the data shows that elementary school boys are more likely to be engaged in being loud, blurting, interrupting, and "inappropriate" climbing and running. It is these kinds of behaviors in school that will get a child flagged for interventions, which is one path toward diagnosis.

Again, I want to point to the question of culture as a factor in the expression of symptoms. Students who don't fit in smoothly with the culture of school get flagged for interventions. The inattentive flavor of ADHD seems to me to be merely the heavily masked form

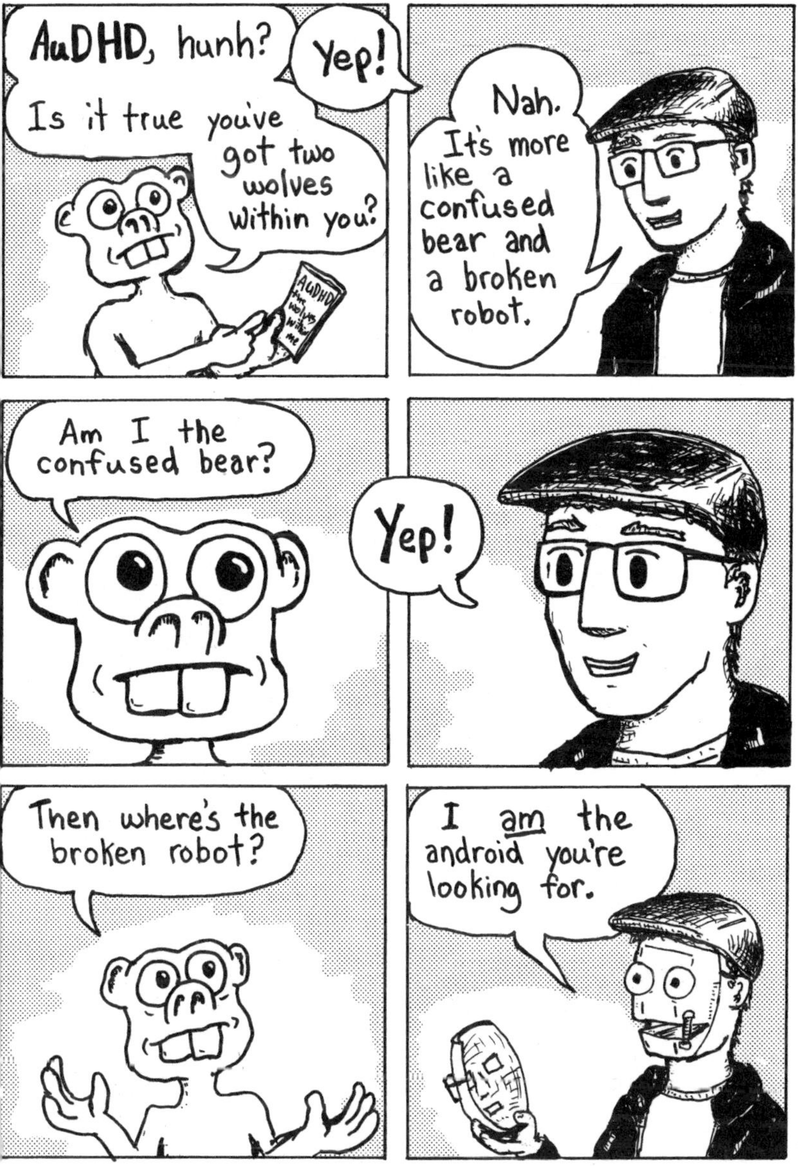
AuDHD, hunh?
Yep!
Is it true you've got two wolves within you?
Nah. It's more like a confused bear and a broken robot.
Am I the confused bear?
Yep!
Then where's the broken robot?
I am the android you're looking for.

of ADHD.

From my firsthand experience, I have seen girls do all the things on the hyperactive-impulsive list. Especially since kids came back to school after the COVID shutdowns. The whole culture of children in America has changed in a way the culture of school hasn't caught up with.

What about transgender/nonbinary children and ADHD?

Yes. A lot of them have ADHD too. Possibly with higher incidence than in cisgender kids. Or maybe neurodivergent kids are more likely to question the validity of the cultural constructs around gender. A definite overlap exists between transgender/nonbinary folx and neurodivergence in general. I really don't want to confuse correlation with causation here. It's entirely possible that people who are more comfortable being open about their gender and sexuality are also more comfortable with being open about things like ADHD.

Is being neurodivergent the same thing as having ADHD?

No. That's like asking if being a mammal is the same thing as being a dog.

What does being neurodivergent mean?

Being neurodivergent means that a person's brain and nervous system work differently than those in the overall majority of people, that majority being referred to as "neurotypicals." In fact, neurodivergent brains work differently in such a way that can be measured in fMRI scans.

Now, there are many varieties of neurodivergence: ADHD, autism, epilepsy, bipolar, Tourette's, OCD, dyslexia, dyspraxia, dyscalculia, dysgraphia, etc. Heck, some people even count left-handedness as a neurodivergence.

A lot of neurodivergence is the result of genetics. Some of it relates to how a developing human responds to factors in the environment, like fetal alcohol exposure or environmental lead poisoning. There is also neurodivergence that has its roots in physical injury or disease, such as a traumatic brain injury or the aftereffects of a severe stroke.

A lot of neurodivergent conditions have debilitating aspects to them that result in neurodivergent people needing different supports to function more fully in the neurotypical world.

Is neurodivergence the same thing as Neurodiversity?

They look so close, don't they? I don't want to be a negative nellie, but, no, they're not the same. In fact, I'm making the stylistic call right here to say the word *Neurodiversity* should be capitalized and *neurodivergent* should remain lowercase to help us remember that they are two different things. While *neurodivergent* is a useful adjective describing a specific subset of human beings, *Neurodiversity* is an all-encompassing ideal. In fact, it's more than an ideal. It's a social justice movement.

The Neurodiversity Movement is a widespread effort to call for and create changes in the neurotypical-dominated social landscape to make it easier for neurodivergent people to have full and rewarding lives. It's about acceptance and accessibility. It's also about working toward providing appropriate supports for people with invisible as well as visible disabilities.

More than anything, the Neurodiversity Movement has the stated goal of including neurodivergent people, voices, and perspectives when making decisions that affect them. The old disability rights slogan still applies: "Nothing about us without us."

Isn't everybody a little bit neurodivergent?

Only in the sense that everybody's a little bit Irish on St. Patrick's Day. By which I mean, no. 80% to 85% of people are neurotypical. Their brains work the way doctors expect the standard human brain to operate. The problem is that neurotypicals love to overgeneralize almost as much as they love being included in things.

(Perhaps we could create a false syllogism with the Irish thing so that neurotypicals can consider themselves a little bit neurodivergent on the Feast Day of St. Bernadette. But only if they make the pilgrimage to Lourdes and . . . no. I take it back. It's a bad joke, and I don't want it becoming a thing.)

What Is AuDHD?

AuDHD is not a diagnostic term. It is a portmanteau of the terms *autistic* and *ADHD*. This is one of those nonmedical terms that emerged from the lived-experience, social-media world as people started getting dually diagnosed as both. This was not a thing that really happened before 2013. The old diagnostic criteria were written in such a way that it led doctors to the opinion that a person could have one condition or the other, but not both.

So, for a long time, whichever set of traits were more prominent would be the ones that got addressed, while the others just magically disappeared because the big, fat book said they didn't exist. And that worked just fine and no one ever got misdiagnosed, misunderstood, or alienated, or developed substance abuse problems or contemplated/acted on suicide.

Disregard that last paragraph. It was all bullshit. Those things happened. Often. And we're trying hard to get over it.

The simple fact is that ADHD and autism definitely co-occur in a significant amount of people. I've seen percentages quoted in a staggering and confusing variety: 17% of the 10% of the population who have ADHD also have autism, while 50% of the 2.8% of people with autism also have ADHD.[4] Do we add those numbers together? Or do we only count the overlap? Either way, my basic arithmetic skills tell me the AuDHD rate is in the 1.7% to 3.1% range. Which

---

4 Camille Hours, Christophe Recasens, and Jean-Marc Baleyte, "ASD And ADHD Comorbidity: What Are We Talking About?", Frontiers in Psychiatry, February 28, 2022, https://doi.org/10.3389/fpsyt.2022.837424.

is confusing, because that's higher than the latest overall autism rate figures from the CDC. Of course, depending on what study you look at, those numbers will shift around more, especially as more and better data is aggregated. Science is really at the early stages of looking into this comorbidity pairing.

What is extra confusing is that some autism traits can look like ADHD traits, and vice versa. Also, one of the fun things about autism is that autistic people don't always respond to medications the same way neurotypical people do. But why keep that fuzziness on the autism side of the line? It is also an observed fact that stimulant medications work differently for ADHDers than they do for neurotypicals. So, from a diagnoser's and a prescriber's perspective, it can be very difficult to tease out which trait is what and which strategy will help.

Ironically, and in the case of myself, the traits of one can mask the traits of the other in a strange, counter-balanced, yin-yang of Neurodiversity that can make you appear to be a perfectly functioning neurotypical for as many as fifteen minutes at a time! In fact, some AuDHDers are so good at masking and compensating because the autistic-distinct anxiety adds a sense of urgency and danger to every single thing you do in the day, which helps keep the ADHD brain engaged.

The good news is, a lot of the everyday strategies for autism and ADHD help out with both. If it turns out that the ADHD stimulant meds help an autistic person function, it's AuDHD. It's not a medical diagnosis. It's just a shorthand for indicating what supports might be helpful for that person. Of course, one of the commonly reported results of an autistic person starting ADHD meds is that they find their autistic traits like hand flapping, toe walking, and social and communication quirks increase while they're getting used to the meds. And they are thrilled that they don't feel that exhausting compulsion to mask their traits so hard. (These are self-reports on social media, so, of course, this information is anecdotal in nature and not hard, researched fact. It's quite possible there is a large and silent AuDHD contingent that hates the fact that they aren't masking as well when they're on Adderall.)

What are all these acronyms and initialisms ADHDers use on social media?

Before I get into it, I want to come right out and say I'm kind of tired of acronyms and initialisms. I worked in education for over fifteen years and had to negotiate an environment full of constantly shifting terminology and hours of PD (professional development) devoted to learning the latest developments in acronyms and initialisms. Very little of it was actually anything now, but people liked to establish their place in the social hierarchy of the faculty and staff by how quickly they could incorporate the new terms into their vocabulary. So, I've learned to be skeptical of the function of initialisms. All too often, they seemed to be used for nothing more than to define who is in-group and who is out-group.

In my opinion, if you want actual meaning to be conveyed, you're better off using actual words.

That being said, language and meaning are constantly shifting. Sometimes, establishing social status is the message. That seems to be what social media is all about, so people pepper their Reels and TikToks with professional, and professional-sounding, terms in a bid to strengthen their message. And then it gets weird when a bunch of people start copying this use of professional terms and language, even though they don't really have a professional-level understanding of what they're talking about. (I'm looking at you, ChatGPT!)

So, of course, people are going to go on social media and label their experiences with acronyms like ACES (adverse childhood experiences), RSD (rejection-sensitive dysphoria), or C-PTSD (complex post-traumatic stress disorder) to justify why they have such a hard time with certain things. But these are all very nuanced concepts that often mean very different things than the influencers touting them say they mean.

I'm not saying these people's experiences aren't real; I'm just saying that the way they toss the terms around is a little cringe for people who have advanced degrees and specialized training in the alphabet soup of diagnostic terms. And some of these terms aren't actually diagnostic terms.

Because I do not have one of these advanced degrees, I'm going to try to not make an ass out of myself using these terms lightly. (While it is very tempting to use RSD because it's an easy shorthand to describe the total plunge into existential nausea I feel when my wife suggests I should wear a different shirt to dinner, am I really using the term right? Can I just use the term "rejection crash" and save myself an awkward email exchange with Dr. Faith? Yeah. I can do that. For the record, the email exchange did happen, and it wasn't that awkward. At least for me.)

ADHD MEDS

The prescription medications for ADHD are literally life changers. One of the biggest checks to see if you really have ADHD is if the ADHD meds are helpful for you. If they aren't, maybe you're struggling with the endemic postmodern, post-COVID VAST traits so many people have picked up from screen life. A lot of strategies for ADHD work well for VAST, but not the meds. For whatever reason, the ADHD meds work differently for ADHDers than they do for neurotypicals.

Okay, it's more than just for whatever reason. There are science reasons, and I'll go into those later. The important thing to note is that the ADHD meds can absolutely help people with ADHD.

My adult daughter was diagnosed several months before I was. (This is often how a neurodivergent diagnosis journey goes. It's in the family.) How she let me know about her new diagnosis was by calling me up and saying, "I never knew doing everyday stuff like folding laundry could actually be enjoyable." Right out of the gate, Adderall was helping her function in tasks she'd been struggling with for decades.

If you've lived with me for any amount of time, you'll know that I also struggle with folding laundry. It helped a little when Marie Kondo showed us how fun folding things can be, but the shiny newness of her techniques wore off pretty quickly. I have to make a conscious effort not to wind up in a chronic floordrobe situation.

When I got diagnosed, I had a couple other monumental self-realization moments. The first one came the day I started taking meds. All year, I'd been having new troubles at my job working in an elementary school. My well-practiced autism strategies were suddenly no longer enough after a new baby entered my life. One area at work that dogged me in particular was whenever I came into a particular third grade classroom. This was a room where I'd already had to diffuse a lot of tense situations. These kids were the COVID Kinder cohort, and they collectively have a lot of trauma they're working on. They are very active, need a lot of attention, interrupt without knowing it, and are prone to large emotional outbursts at the drop of a hat. (Basically, they're a case study for VAST prevalence among elementary school children.) At a certain point during the school year, I became very aware that I hardly ever knew what the teacher's instructions were in that room. I blamed the atmosphere of chaos, my advancing age, and my auditory processing issues. At one point, I directed my frustration towards the fact that there were so many colorful posters up on the walls. Basically, I was pegging the problem on so many variables I couldn't control and felt terribly helpless in the situation.

The very first day I had my ADHD meds, I could track every instruction the teacher gave. It was a miracle. A little tweak of chemistry helped me get through the rest of the school year.

I don't want to imply that every ADHDer needs meds to function. I go into this more a little further down, but I want to say up front that, while the meds can be very helpful, there are many reasons why they may not be the best strategy depending on the individual. The meds can be a very powerful tool, but they aren't the only tool. However, to safely use this tool, you need a medical diagnosis.

How does someone get a diagnosis?

There are many paths to diagnosis. And, like all things ADHD, it might take a few attempts to find the right path for you. Also, my sphere of knowledge is limited to how things work in the United States, so, as with all things ADHD, results may vary

A good starting point is talking to your regular doctor, your primary care physician. They can, hopefully, get you a referral to a knowledgeable diagnosing clinician. If you don't have a regular doctor, or you are in an iffy health insurance situation, there might be a few more steps in your way on this path.

(I don't want to heap shame on anyone for not having health insurance. The American healthcare system is built from a hodgepodge of seemingly contradictory laws and is administered by an uncoordinated mix of for-profit, nonprofit, not-for-profit, and governmental entities. There are many opportunities for the system to fail, and it does.)

If you already have a regular therapist you see, you could bring up your ADHD questions with them. In fact, prepare yourself to stay on track for this conversation by bringing with you a filled-out ASRS (Adult ADHD Self-Report Screening) form. It's freely available in multiple places online. Just search "Adult ADHD Self-Report."

But, also, be prepared for the fact that therapists have their specialties that they are very, very good at. Not all of them are very, very good at ADHD. If your therapist responds using old diagnostic terminology, like ADD, or suggests that you're too old to be diagnosed, these are signs that you should find someone else to take your ADHD-specific questions to.

(One note on terminology: The terms *neurodivergent* and *Neurodiversity* come from outside the medical and psychological professions. If a therapist doesn't seem comfortable with using these terms in a clinical setting, it might not be a total red flag. Their training just hasn't caught up with the language the Neurodiversity Movement likes to use.)

There is also the self-diagnosis path. I think most adult-identified ADHDers take a stroll along this path in the beginning. Self-diagnosis involves doing a lot of reading up on the subject. Taking online assessments. Talking to people who have diagnoses. Comparing stories. Basically, self-diagnosis is taking a read on whether your personal experiences match up with those of people who have medical diagnoses. You also get a chance to try the little tips and hacks they have to share.

I basically came to my self-diagnosis stage in a backward way. I started listening to ADHDers talk about things that helped them out, and I tried them. It wasn't until later that I put together, *Oh, these ADHD life hacks work for me because I have ADHD.*

And then there is the telemedicine path. There are several companies out there that offer online diagnostic tools of varying legitimacy. A lot of times, the diagnosis portion is a precursor to starting a subscription to whatever remedy they are selling. Some of them are selling "proprietary blends" of herbal supplements. Some of them are prescription mills for stimulant medications. A lot of them aren't covered by health insurance, which, in the case of mail-order Schedule II prescription medications, gives me the gut feel that what's going on isn't entirely ethical.

This is not to discount telemedicine visits with providers altogether. I'm just very skeptical about the ones without a lot of transparency about how they operate. In the case of Done Global Inc., the DEA is also skeptical.

Should everyone with ADHD be on ADHD meds?

No. Everyone's overall medical situation is different. Very often, ADHD is not the only medical concern a person has. Some of the medications can have interactions with other medications. The medications are designed to change the levels of certain hormones in the body. If you have another medical condition that requires management of hormone levels, like diabetes, the ADHD drugs may cause more problems than they solve.

In my own experience, while I don't have diabetes, since I started taking Adderall, my body responds differently to highly-processed sugar. I have to watch it when I eat desserts or pastries made with

Side Quest:

The Self-Diagnosis Debate

There are a lot of differing opinions on the validity of self-diagnosis.

From the social model of disability standpoint, sometimes the access to a medical diagnosis has a ridiculous amount of barriers. It can take a long time to get an appointment with a diagnosing clinician. In some countries, the waitlist is years long. In the U.S., there might be problems finding a good provider who takes your health insurance. Just managing to make a phone call, let alone schedule an appointment, can be a dealbreaker for someone with ADHD. So, until those barriers to a formal diagnosis can be overcome, self-diagnosis might be the only realistic option for a while.

From the medical model point of view, self-diagnosis is dangerous. There is the possibility that other serious conditions with similar symptoms will go untreated. Also, you can't get medication without a medical diagnosis and a prescription. So, self-diagnosed folx may be more likely to self-medicate with substances from less reputable sources. Danger aside, there is also the legal angle. In order to be covered by the legal protections for people with disabilities, you need a formal diagnosis.

There are other points of contention in the self-diagnosis debate, but most of them seem like they come from people who really like arguing on the internet. It's hard for me to parse out what the substance of these arguments are, beyond some people wanting to establish that they are either as valid, or more valid, than other people. I don't find that kind of discourse that helpful, so I move on.

an American-level of sweetness. I am liable to get very wound up and start yelling at people about astronomy. (Nobody wants this. No more glazed donuts for me.)

And figuring out which meds work best? And which dose you need? That's a very individual process. My adult daughter, an ADHDer, is also my go-to expert on being self-aware of how medications actually affect you (she has some scary rehab stories, and speaks from experience). On her holiday visit a little over a year ago, she kindly suggested that my dose might be a little too high based on how annoyingly excited I was at nine in the morning. (Touché, Star. Touché.) Which is why it is good to have good relationships with people who know you very well. The medications, when they work, shouldn't transform your personality.

And this is tricky in the case of kids. Do younger kids, who don't even know who they are yet, get a valid benefit from the medication?

Sometimes yes, sometimes no, and sometimes it's the wrong med. Results will vary, and they will especially vary over time as those younger bodies grow and change. And by change, I do include puberty, and all the variations thereof.

Why is it easier to get meds prescribed in some countries than in others?

In one sense, it's cultural. In another sense, it's business.

In the United States of America, the dominant culture is business. As an American, I live in a very pharmaceutical-forward country. Culturally, Americans would rather purchase a quick fix than actually do some work to fix things properly. As evidence, I will shrug vaguely at the opioid crisis dumpster fire around me.

The U.S. healthcare system has this problem baked into it. The managers of health plans have decided it can be more cost effective for them to try medications first and hope that solves it. In the case of ADHD, the meds can do a good deal of the heavy lifting to help someone get to the point where they can start applying external and behavioral strategies to their lives. So, while other countries will spend more time and resources on those other interventions first, it can take longer to get to the pharmaceutical intervention.

Which is right and which is wrong? I couldn't tell you. Everyone is on a different journey. And those journeys are heavily flavored by the cultural, political, and economic landscape each person finds themselves in.

What are the medications for ADHD?

There are three basic categories of meds that are effective: stimulants, stimulant-like drugs, and the miscellaneous outlier category of other drugs that help for some reason. Listing them in order seems kind of boring to me, so I'm going to do a countdown instead.

At number three, outlier drugs are things that, surprise, help with the co-occuring issues with ADHD. One of the big problems ADHDers face is this newly-named thing called rejection-sensitive dysphoria (RSD), which a couple old-school blood pressure meds like clonidine can really help with. (Faith chimed in with a note that these meds have an effect on impulse control, which is why they also are handy for people quitting smoking.)The outlier drugs may be used on their own, or in combination with other ADHD meds.

Coming in at number two, we have the stimulant-like drugs, which act to boost the same brain chemicals that stimulants do, but do so through different mechanisms than the stimulants do. Wellbutrin is one of these that I've seen some commercials for as something to help depression, in addition to the old SSRIs. It takes a while longer for the stimulant-like drug to build up to full strength, but there's different risks associated with them.

And, finally, the number one, all-time champion category at helping the ADHD brain get over the hump of managing daily life is stimulant medication. The stimulants do a great job of releasing the important brain chemicals of dopamine and norepinephrine. These are the exact chemicals the ADHD brain is constantly running low on over the course of the day. Within the stimulants category, there are two basic types of drugs: the methylphenidate type (think Ritalin) and the amphetamine type (think Adderall).

Aren't amphetamines things Nancy Reagan wanted us to just say no to?

I know. Crazy, right? Both the methylphenidate and amphetamine drugs are Schedule II controlled substances in the United States. There are warnings against abuse and addiction associated with them. So, understandably, there is a worry about taking these drugs or, shock, giving them to children. Especially after the propaganda we've been fed by the long-standing War on Drugs in the United States.

So, let's dial back the paranoia for a moment.

First of all, your current prescription grade Adderall XR is generations more refined than the over the counter Benzedrine that Jack Kerouac powered down to type out *On the Road* in a sleepless, three-week binge. There has been plenty of research and product history to back up the fact that the properly prescribed dosage and formulation of today's ADHD medications are very safe. There is also plenty of data backing up the fact that ADHD brains respond to stimulant medication very differently than neurotypical recreational users.

That being said, it's entirely possible that Jack Kerouac got into amphetamines and coffee as a way to self-medicate ADHD in the days before it was recognized. I'm sure a lot of people did. But I'm not in the business of handing out posthumous diagnoses to historical figures. I'm just saying it wouldn't surprise me.

Getting back to what I do know, the stimulant drugs used to treat ADHD are very controlled. Fine-tuning the dosage and which drug works best for an individual takes time and close cooperation with the prescriber. There are no automatic refills at the pharmacy.

The doctor has to call it in every time. And if you've signed up for an online service that sends you ADHD meds in the mail on regular schedule for a higher price than your normal prescription copay, you might actually be supporting an unethical or illegal business operation like Done Global Inc., which, as of this writing, has just been majorly busted.

And, while we're on the topic of illegal and unethical business operations, it is highly recommended that you do not seek out street sources of ADHD meds. You don't know what you're really getting and the dosage control isn't there. And while, yes, there is a prescription version of methamphetamine that is sometimes prescribed for ADHD, for glob's sake, don't get ice on the street and think it'll be good for you. One of the problems with methamphetamine, especially in the kind of high doses you'll find in street versions, is that it is actually toxic to the dopaminergic pathways in the brain that already need extra help in ADHD brains.

Also, these days, fentanyl is all over the place in your street versions of pharmaceutical products. Fentanyl is not a drug you want to mess around with the dosage of. It works great in the hospital in very controlled doses. Licensed anesthesiologists are very good at their jobs. Street level "pharmaceutical reps," not so much. When fentanyl is used as a cheap filler in party drugs, young people die. Also, for people in the Borderlands who like to get their prescriptions filled at a discount in Mexico, look out. Lots of counterfeits enter the marketplace in places markets aren't as highly regulated. And these days, those counterfeits are often laced with fentanyl. So, best practice to keep yourself alive is to get the ADHD meds through licensed and regulated channels.

How do the meds work?

The stimulant drugs increase the amount of dopamine and norepinephrine present in the brain. These are important brain molecules, or neurotransmitters, that help keep things running smoothly. Dopamine is associated with several pathways in the brain, one of them being highly involved with motivation. Norepinephrine is produced in the adrenal glands and prods the central nervous system into arousal, alertness, and being ready to act. Having more of these chemicals present helps the whole central nervous system work better. Remember the glitchy switches between the TPN and the DMN networks in the brain? Dopamine and norepinephrine help those switches not be so glitchy.

The ADHD brain has trouble producing enough dopamine and norepinephrine during most situations. The methylphenidate-based drugs like Ritalin prevent your system from reabsorbing the dopamine and norepinephrine too quickly. Amphetamine-based drugs like Adderall work, in part, by causing your brain to release more dopamine and norepinephrine.

There are times when the ADHD brain does produce these neurotransmitters pretty well: when there's a sense of urgency, excitement, or impending danger. This is probably why kids with ADHD like climbing on stuff they're not supposed to climb on. The thrill of defying gravity! It's also why I had a hell of a time towards the end of every semester in college. All of the big research papers were coming due and I hadn't been able to get a start on them until the dreaded urgency of a looming deadline kicked in.

Having the meds support your nervous system makes it so an ADHDer can actually get started on something without the fear of injury, death, bad grades, or getting fired (although sometimes we'd actually prefer being fired).

Why are there different types of meds?

Because everybody's a little different. Our own bodies react differently to medications. With a lot of medications, that window of effectiveness is big enough for most people. Over-the-counter pain relievers do a pretty good job most of the time for most people. That being said, acetaminophen is one of the most commonly overdosed drugs.

The over-the-counter analog for stimulant drugs would be caffeine. The world runs on coffee. But, also, I can drink a cup of coffee at four in the afternoon and immediately take a nap.

If you need something more than the recommended dose of Tylenol, or more than a cup of coffee to get you going, getting a doctor's involvement is key. Prescription medications require more fine-tuning to the individual. It can take a while to find the right dosage and the right medicine. Some people respond better to the methylphenidate-type meds (like Ritalin) than the amphetamine-type (Adderall). There are also immediate release and extended release (XR) versions. It can take some trial and error to determine what works best for the individual. And, of course, drug efficacy changes over time as tolerances are built up.

Do the meds work the same for men and women?

So, big picture, the meds work differently individual to individual. Getting more granular, and considering how many people look at gender as a social construct, this question can take us down a whole lot of rabbit holes. So, to keep us on track, I'm going to go with AFAB (assigned female at birth) and AMAB (assigned male at birth) as our starting point.

Because the drugs work by changing the levels of neurotransmitters in the brain, they can get some competing interference with other factors that change levels of neurotransmitters in the brain. Brains in AMAB bodies, for the most part, don't have the same fluctuations in hormones as AFAB bodies. There's the big change at adolescence, then a plateau for about fifteen to twenty years, followed by a slow decline over the remaining decades of the AMAB body's existence.

After the tumult of puberty is over, AFAB bodies, generally, go through cyclical hormone changes that affect neurotransmitters every month, with different changes that happen during pregnancy, childbirth, and breastfeeding. Then there's perimenopause, which can be as impactful as, or more impactful than, puberty, in terms

ADHD Meds

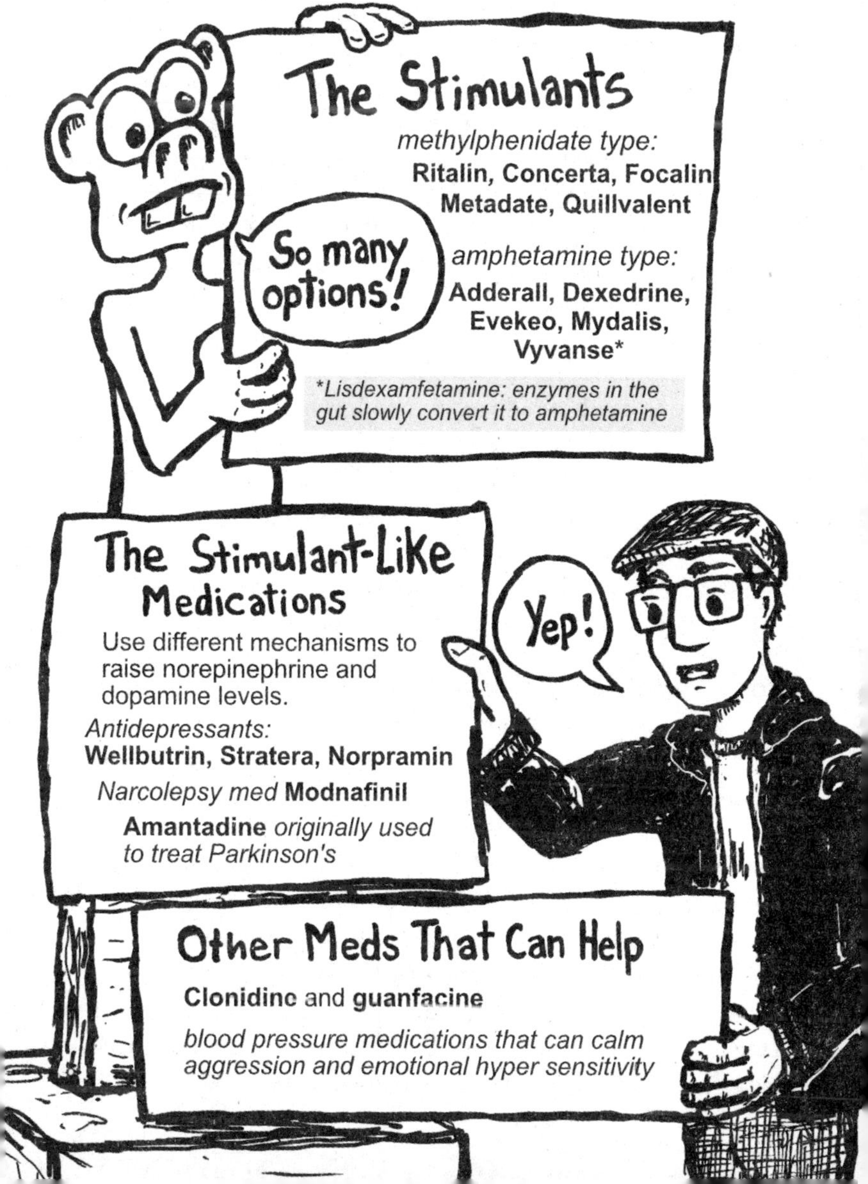
The Stimulants
methylphenidate type:
Ritalin, Concerta, Focalin
Metadate, Quillvalent
amphetamine type:
Adderall, Dexedrine,
Evekeo, Mydalis,
Vyvanse*
*Lisdexamfetamine: enzymes in the gut slowly convert it to amphetamine
So many options!
The Stimulant-Like Medications
Use different mechanisms to raise norepinephrine and dopamine levels.
Antidepressants:
Wellbutrin, Stratera, Norpramin
Narcolepsy med Modnafinil
Amantadine originally used to treat Parkinson's
Yep!
Other Meds That Can Help
Clonidine and guanfacine
blood pressure medications that can calm aggression and emotional hyper sensitivity

of hormone fluctuations that affect neurotransmitters. AFAB bodies don't really get a break until after menopause.

Many AFAB ADHDers have stated a very strong desire to have flexibility to adjust their dosage according to the needs of their bodies during these natural fluctuations. And yet doctors, the FDA, and the DEA insist on dispensing the stimulant meds to women on the same constrained dosage schedules that only really make sense for prepubescent children and AMAB bodies.

That only covers one chunk of the whole spectrum of gender and biological sex presentation and how they interact with what's going on in the brain. I'm going to have to admit that there's a lot I don't know, because my lived experience is limited to my own mildly gender-nonconforming AMAB life. That said, from a standpoint of advocating for Neurodiversity and inclusion, I believe that the medical establishment has a lot of work to do towards taking into account and accommodating the experiences of people who don't fit the parameters of the models they've been given to work with. It makes intuitive sense to me that trans, intersex, and nonbinary people are going to have some concerns and issues that don't mesh with the standard models of how the meds work.

What are the side effects of ADHD meds?

This is a question with a potentially huge answer. If you watch any sort of television with advertising, you're probably familiar with the hushed tones of the long legal disclaimers listing all the known possible side effects of whatever drug they're selling. And, invariably, those disclaimers include risks of diarrhea and potentially fatal blood clots.

So, I could give you the deep dive legal disclaimer list, or I can tell you what I think is the most useful information for you to get before you talk to your doctor. The most common side effects are decreased appetite, weight loss, and trouble sleeping. Usually these side effects lessen as your body gets used to the medication. There are also some modifications you can make to your life to alleviate these, including the following:

- Eating a good meal before you take your first dose of the day.
- Choosing highly nutritious foods so your body can get what it needs with smaller meals.
- Taking your meds early enough in the day that they'll wear off before bedtime
- Saving the megadose vitamin C for an hour or two before bed, if you take vitamin supplements. Vitamin C likes to snatch the stimulant meds out of the bloodstream and send them straight to your urinary system.

Other common and less pleasant side effects are upset stomach, anxiety, and changes in blood pressure and heart rate. If you're starting ADHD meds and you're having new trouble in these areas, definitely talk to your doctor. It may be the kind of thing a change in dosage or in medication will help. Also, you don't want to mess around with cardiac issues. My doctor made sure I had a clean EKG before even giving me a prescription.

Another side effect is the rebound effect. I'm a rebounder myself. This just means when the meds wear off, I get a short period of fatigue. This usually hits me in the mid-afternoon, at a time when I tend to have low energy anyway. If I can get away with taking a nap, no problem. If I can't nap, it's not unmanageable. I just give myself grace for about an hour while my brain recharges. Other people may experience a drop in mood during the rebound period. It follows that a sudden drop in energy can correspond with a bad mood. It probably helps that, as a maturing Gen Xer, I've had enough real life experience to know that a cranky afternoon does not have to become a cranky rest of the day.

Some people—and this may sound absolutely unreasonable, but

I've seen them do it—some people get in a bit of cardio exercise to rev up some endorphins. Or some people have a low-dose, midday boost of the non-XR meds. The trick to that strategy is that it can be very easy to forget to take that midday dose. There's a lot of personal nuance to getting through the afternoon lull. In practice, I have learned that, if I don't want to take a nap, I shouldn't lie down.

Something else to look out for with the ADHD meds is how they may interact with other medications you take. This is another reason to make sure you have a good, honest relationship with your doctor—not just taking one of your little cousin's pills to see what it does. One of these people has a professional and legal interest in making sure you don't have an avoidable high blood pressure crisis.

Do the ADHD meds help with executive function?

Yes and no. The stimulant medications do a really good job helping the ADHD brain focus on things. However, they don't help you pick which things to focus on. So, if you have other tools and strategies in place, the meds can help you stay on track.

For example, if I have a straightforward schedule or to-do list ready to go for the day, the meds will help me stick to the items on that list . . . so long as I don't lose the list or put it somewhere I can't easily refer to it. The meds do a great job of helping your brain filter out environmental or social noise that might make it hard to stay on schedule.

However, every interruption to the schedule or list is an opportunity for focus to be directed elsewhere. And these opportunities are decision points where we need our executive function to kick in and help us make a choice about which path we take: the scheduled path, or the shiny new interruption.

Without the meds, we might spin aimlessly in indecision for minutes, or hours, trying to figure out how to deal with the interruption. With the meds, we can make that decision almost immediately. But, without other tools and strategies in place, there's

Side Quest:

Side Effects

Multiple neurodivergent people might notice some interesting things when they start ADHD meds. There have been a lot of anecdotal reports from autistic people who start taking meds after being newly identified as also ADHD. Many describe a sudden inability to put on their social masks. Autistic masking is a monumental experience that deserves its own book. So, cutting to the chase, something about the ADHD meds makes it easier for autistic people to relax into their unmasked state when around others. What this means is there's a good chance that long-suppressed tics, flaps, blurts, toe walking, echolalia, scripting, and autistic joy spasms are going to start coming out more when the AuDHDer starts their meds. Especially if these are the kinds of things they like to do when they are feeling good about themselves

Again, a lot to unpack, and it deserves a lot more than I can give it in this sidebar.

There have also been some studies that suggest ADHD meds have a positive effect on dyslexic student's reading scores. Have there been enough studies? Are the subjects of these studies officially diagnosed with both ADHD and dyslexia? How many variables can we actually control for in these studies?

Having worked in education, I'm very hesitant to jump in on this one as it's not clear to me where correlation and causation begin and end here. There are so many factors at play.

But the anecdotals on the AuDHDers are very interesting to me because a week into taking Adderall, I caught myself toe walking again. A few months later, I find consistently that I'm not rattled as much by sensory overwhelm in social situations. Which can manifest as both not needing to stim as much *and* not caring as much if the stimming might seem odd to those around me. So, at this point, it seems to be a twofer.

still a really good chance we'll pick doing the shiny new thing over doing the thing that puts supper on the table in time.

Are meds enough to treat ADHD without using other strategies?

No. The meds can help a lot, but they don't solve all the problems. Like usual, if you want to solve problems, you have to do some work. Ideally, the meds help you focus on that work. But the meds can also really help you focus on scrolling through TikTok for a couple hours before you suddenly get a calendar reminder of an important event happening in thirty minutes. Do you have enough time to get ready? Or would it have been helpful to have some more structural things in place to get you out the door in time?

Also, it's really good to have some strategies in place to help you keep going when you can't fill your prescription due to shortages.

Wait a minute. There are shortages?

Yes. As of this writing, my prescription is on back order. Luckily, I have a bit of a cushion. I'm new to the meds, I've kept my dose low, and I've been intentionally taking "vacation" days to keep the meds effective and give my system a chance to rest. (Knowing myself, I know a little bit of medication can quickly take me way too far if I'm not careful. This is probably more related to my autism traits than the ADHD.)

Why are there shortages?

The stimulant medications that are very effective at helping ADHDers are Schedule II controlled substances in the United States. They are similarly controlled in many other countries. As such, the production, prescription, and distribution of these medications is heavily regulated by the FDA and the DEA. The manufacturers literally need to get government approval for every batch they make.

So, that's one layer of complication in the supply.

The next layer is the good old capitalistic mechanism of supply and demand. Increased awareness and diagnosis of ADHD is increasing the legitimate demand for these medications, while the FDA is trying to regulate the amount of the supply based on outdated diagnosis numbers. At the same time, pharmacy benefit managers are doing their magic to manipulate prices to their benefit as best they can within the constraints of the law.

And then there's the illegitimate demand for these drugs. There are a lot of off-label reasons people use them. Starting with what should be obvious: a lot of people turn to less-than-legal methods to self-medicate conditions they suffer from but haven't gotten formal medical treatment for because there can be a lot of barriers to getting to a proper doctor. The American healthcare system be like that. Unfortunately, not having an educated and licensed physician guide you on which medications and which dosages work well for your specific body and brain can lead to developing a substance abuse problem. (There's a reason they're Schedule II.)

Another form of illegitimate use is by people who take stimulants as a study drug and those who take them to party harder on the weekends. These are often the same people. They are often college students flush with their parents' money. Traditionally, a college student with money can usually find another, poorer college student with some interesting prescription medications that they might be willing to skip a couple doses of. The forces of capitalism work their magic in the gray areas of the free market.

And where there's a market, there is financial adventurism. The COVID-era expansion of telemedicine created new opportunities for business startups. One example is Done Global, which has recently come under scrutiny from the DEA. The founder and the president were both arrested on fraud charges in June 2024.[5] Done Global is

5 Chris Larson, "Done Global Arrests Will Cast a Long Shadow on Behavioral Health," Behavioral Health Business, June 27, 2024, https://bhbusiness.com/2024/06/27/done-global-arrests-will-cast-a-long-shadow-on-behavioral-health/.

one of many companies offering easy, convenient, online ADHD diagnoses and accompanying prescription medication. Many of the rules in place for monitoring these prescriptions have been skirted, or outright ignored, in favor of being able to quickly deliver prescription stimulants at inflated prices. This, combined with the fact that some recreational drug users are turning away from prescription opioids, due to increasing ODs from fentanyl contamination of counterfeit pills. Prescription stimulants seem like a safer bet, especially since there are online telemedicine drug dealers ready to write customers some scrip after a multiple choice assessment quiz and barely any real-time contact with the prescriber.

This has created even more demand for a limited supply. And because the DEA is having trouble figuring out how to assess what the legitimate market is, and how to make sure the drugs legitimately get there, the rich kids are going to get their party drugs, while the rest of us get messages from the pharmacy that our Adderall XR is on back order.

Why does my doctor tell me to NOT take my meds a couple days a week?

Some doctors will specifically advise to take break days, or to skip the meds on weekends. Some of these doctors will only write a prescription for a twenty-eight-day supply. And the pharmacies are legally prohibited from filling the Schedule II drug prescriptions more often than once every thirty days. So, a lot of ADHDers who take the stimulant meds are kind of forced into taking at least two break days a month. And don't be surprised if your doctor wants you to take a drug test before writing your prescription.

You can get mad at the doctors and you can get mad at the government. You can rage and whinge on your social media platform of choice, but it's probably not going to change anything. Maybe you can switch doctors. The Feds really frown on people doctor-shopping for controlled substance prescriptions, so try not to do that any more often than you have to.

The frustrating reality is that the doctors do this because they actually care about your health. It's not necessarily that they're worried about how the meds can become habit-forming for recreational users. They are more concerned your body will build up a tolerance for your meds in a way that can make your dosage less effective over time. This happens with lots of kinds of medications. They are also a little worried about the cardiovascular effects of long-term use.

Of course, the studies that indicate this don't take into account all of the other habits ADHDers tend to pick up that also put wear and tear on the cardiovascular system. So, it's not a given that correlation means causation here.

In any case, because the stimulant meds are something some ADHDers will need for most of their lives, the doctors want to make sure the effective dose for each individual stays as low as possible for as long as possible. For this reason, it is actually a good idea to take breaks. Another reason it's a good idea to take breaks is that it allows you to build up a stockpile for when another one of those dreaded shortages hits.

While the doctors like to suggest taking the break on the weekends, a lot of ADHDers don't have weeks that work like that. Some of us are hustling our second and third jobs. Or, the weekends have social or family demands that are actually easier to handle when we aren't on a break day. When my cousin, who's also AuDHD, found out my doctor recommended I not take the meds on the weekend, he thought that was preposterous. His thought was that he especially wants to be able to function his best when he's on his own time on his days off from work. It's a fair point. Another friend of mine told me that she'll skip the meds on days she knows she won't have to think so hard.

Personally, I've found that by day three or four, I start having trouble sleeping and am more likely to start pointless arguments on the internet and in group text chats. (Like that time I got a stick up my butt about the pronunciation of *Uranus*. I was not correct and have apologized to all involved parties.) I take these things as a little sign that my brain's ready for a reset. I try to catch it before I do anything too damaging. Four days on/one day off seems to be the sweet spot for me right now.

For the record, I'm taking a break day as I'm writing this. So, it's not like your life is totally ruined when you miss your meds for a day. It's harder, but still doable. But it does help to be mindful and adjust your expectations for yourself accordingly. Unfortunately, when the shortages get bad, it can be weeks or months until the pharmacy is able to fill the prescription. Again, it's doable, but gets more exhausting as the days pass. If you have a buffer of unused, break-day pills built up, you can ration them to ease your way through the shortage.

Are controlled ADHD meds addictive and harmful?

There are so many levels of irony to this question.

The first being that one of the big problems ADHDers face is remembering to take their meds. This is especially true of the immediate release formulations that need to be taken multiple times a day. Taking a pill when you wake up? Not so hard to remember. Taking another one four hours later when the first one wears off? Super hard. It's so easy to miss that second dose, especially when the time-blindness kicks in.

The second irony is the reality of living with ADHD med shortages. ADHDers are more likely to skip a dose from time to time in order to build up a cushion in case their regular refill gets back-ordered, than to go nuts and overdo it with the meds.

The third, and most amazing irony is that the ADHD stimulant drugs do not have the same effect on ADHDers as they do on neurotypicals.

Before 1959, amphetamine drugs like Benzedrine were over-the-counter. An early formulation was sold as a nasal decongestant. They've been packaged as diet drugs and pep pills. They were also used as "performance enhancers" by poets, writers, musicians, and mathematicians. Before 1970 and the creation of the DEA's schedule of controlled substances, the biggest complaint about amphetamines was that the people who overused them tended to become ridiculously self-centered and very annoying at parties.[6] So stimulants became unfashionable and marijuana and heroin became cool.

There is a concern about cardiac function, but the long-term data on people who use the stimulant drugs for ADHD shows that there really isn't anything to worry about. Especially when there is so much data on how much more prone to accidental injury and suicide ADHDers are. Russell Barkley, PhD, in a 2020 interview in the *Carlat Child Psychiatry Report* refers to his research that shows "about two-thirds of people with ADHD having a life expectancy reduced by up to twenty-one years."

This is a scary huge figure. I don't exactly know how Barkley crunched the numbers, and, since I'm more of a lived-experience writer than a hard academic, I would probably spend weeks trying to remember how statistics work in order to understand it better. But nobody picked up this book to watch me struggle with math. So, let's cut to the chase. It is basically a no-brainer. The risks of doing nothing to manage a person's ADHD struggles far outweigh the risks associated with taking the right dose of the right medication.

Is there a version of ADHD medication that's less likely to be abused?

Yes. There's the drug lisdexamfetamine, commonly known by the

6 Alan Jacobs, "The Lost World of Benzedrine," The Atlantic, April 16, 2012, https://www.theatlantic.com/health/archive/2012/04/the-lost-world-of-benzedrine/255904/.

brand name Vyvanse, which is actually a chemical that the body metabolizes into dextroamphetamine, the main active ingredient in amphetamine salts. Because it takes the body's biological processes to release the active ingredient, it is delivered slowly and evenly over an extended period of time. The effects kick in about two hours after ingestion and last for twelve hours after that.

If a person were to crunch up and snort lisdexamfetamine, they would not be getting the kind of fun they were looking for. (So don't do this!)

Why do my pain meds work better when I am medicated for my ADHD?

This question came from one of my daily social media research dives, but it hit me hard. Like many neurodivergent folx, I've had periods of chronic pain in my life. It's not fun, and a lot of times the pain meds only do so much.

Before I start getting into my own thoughts, I have to start with the standard caveat: discuss with your doctor all the meds you take and how they can interact with each other.

A quick search of the old NIH's medical library turned up a couple anecdotals about this phenomenon being reported, but no studies into the how and the why.

Based on my experience of having a decade of chronic neck pain immediately vanish when an impacted wisdom tooth was removed in my thirties, I've got a basic theory that goes like this: everything in this body is connected to everything else. Helping one area that's having trouble can have a spillover effect that helps other trouble areas feel better too.

My theory is pretty vague and woo-woo, so I checked in with Dr. Faith Harper to see if she had any more specific knowledge on the topic. She says,

> "ADHD meds stimulate the entire central nervous system. And while I haven't seen any research on the topic, other

clinical nutritionists have had the same experience that I have had that when we support the nervous system, other medications work better too. I explain to clients that when you're ill, the whole system constricts in pain and the meds struggle to get in and work. I've seen kids avoid ear tubes when adding kava to their antibiotic regimens, for example. The meds started working once the nervous system was no longer acting like a heart in V-fib and was relaxed enough for healing to happen."

If you've read any of Faith's books (highly recommended), you'll know that helping that central nervous system function helps with just about everything else.

Are there herbal alternatives to ADHD meds?

I'm going to have to say maybe. Herbal remedies are often not as well-researched as chemical pharmaceuticals. For example, there are a lot of people who tout the benefits of CBD. There's a ton of anecdotal evidence available at the health food store. I have personally enjoyed the calming effects of CBD in the same way I often enjoy an extra gnarly, hopped-up IPA.

Is this CBD enjoyment addressing ADHD symptoms? I really don't know. Some people swear by it. There is some consensus that it really helps the anxiety that tends to go hand in hand with so many neurodivergent conditions.

CBD is, of course, derived from the cannabis plant. It is not the same chemical as the THC from marijuana, although the two do work together as buddy chemicals. It is almost impossible to find a CBD supplement that does not contain trace amounts of THC. This trace amount is nothing to worry about. However, if you have one of those jobs that makes you pee test for drugs, Dr. Faith recommends using CBD that's derived from hemp root only. "Most other versions will make you pop hot for cannabis," she says.

THC, on the other hand—in the higher doses that are used for pain relief, counteracting chemotherapy symptoms, and recreational purposes—really works against all the strategies for proactively managing ADHD. Because of this, my professional brain care person strongly recommended avoiding THC. This wasn't a problem for me, because before that particular consultation, I had exactly one experience with a THC gummy. I can tell you this much: the most noticeable effect for me was that I could not pay attention to anything. I hated that feeling of losing my grasp on something I work so hard at doing. I don't see myself trying THC again.

ADHDer comics artist Zuzu (@ZuZu_Cartoons) recommended a brand of mushroom-infused coffee to me for help with staying focused on drawing for a couple hours at a time. I tried this before I got my ADHD diagnosis, and I tell you what, that coffee mixed with lion's mane helps keep my butt in the chair when I'm drawing stuff.

Again, Dr. Faith, my friend with clinical nutritionist training, let me know a lot of clinical nutritionists like to use what she calls "grounding minerals," like magnesium or zinc supplements, to help ADHDers. She's also seen some success with dessicated adrenal support for ADHDers for whom the meds "kick in kinda hard, and the adrenal support makes the transition easier."

Another big name in the supplements aisle at the health food store is ginkgo biloba. Ginkgo biloba extract is derived from a living dinosaur of a tree that has been cultivated by humans in Asia for thousands of years. It has been used to support cognitive function for ages. It's a go-to herbal supplement for anything brain-related and has minimal side effects. The big warning is that it can have adverse interactions with other medications, especially with anticoagulants, and it may trigger seizures in people with seizure disorders. Some studies have shown that ginkgo, when taken in combination with methylphenidate drugs, increases attention in children with ADHD. It doesn't seem to help with hyperactivity or impulsiveness, just attentiveness. Also, these studies were done on children with the behavioral data reported by teachers and parents. I'm curious to hear what results adult ADHDers have experienced with ginkgo.

There are lots of other herbal supplements out there. Some of them do some good central nervous system support. Some of them, like ginkgo biloba and lion's mane, have been used in traditional Asian medicine for centuries. I hope I don't have to explain that western medical science has a bias against traditional remedies that extends to not doing too much research into them. Most pharmaceutical research is funded by big drug companies in the hopes of being able to cash in for seventeen years on an exclusive patent. They're not that interested in finding out if some mushroom you can find at H-Mart does as good a job for cheaper. I think there's something to be said for looking into something that has centuries of tradition behind it. Especially if it doesn't come at the expense of an endangered species. (The patent for Viagra expired a while ago. The generic is cheap. There's no need to harvest rhino horns to make boner pills.)

Some may argue that herbal supplements only work because of the placebo effect. But, hey, sometimes the placebo effect is your friend. Either way, if something is helpful, it's helpful. That being said, I have to insist on the importance of consulting with your doctor about the herbal supplements you take. We don't want any unwanted side effects or harmful interactions.

What about that new alternative product I saw an online ad for?

Well, if it's the same product *I* saw an ad for, I couldn't get any information about what's in it without giving the company a bunch of personal information. So, I'm naturally skeptical. First off, I don't like it when a company exploits the information differential between themselves and their customers. Right away, that tells me they are more interested in making a sale than providing a good product. More importantly, if I don't know what the ingredients are, I can't look to my trusted resources to find out if they're bullshit or not. So, I can't recommend it.

What about vitamin and mineral supplements?

In general, you want to maintain good nutrition. I know that's hard with the ADHD gremlins constantly hijacking your meal-planning abilities. It is very difficult for me to prepare food for myself that involves more than three steps. This can make getting the right nutrients from food an iffy proposition.

In general, a daily multivitamin is not a bad idea. Vitamin D, B complex, magnesium, zinc, calcium, and vitamin C are all great for keeping the brain and body maintained. If there are vitamins or minerals you know you are deficient in (because the doctor saw this indicated in your bloodwork), by all means take them. Also, your doctor may know if there's a specific-to-you reason not to take a certain supplement.

One important thing to note is that vitamin C can interact with ADHD meds in an unhelpful, but not dangerous, way. It basically breaks down and removes the medication from your bloodstream before it has a chance to do you any good. So save the vitamin C for later in your day.

NON-MEDICATION ADHD STRATEGIES

Good news! There are plenty of these, and they are really useful.

It is my opinion that, with ADHD being as common as left-handedness, it is probably nothing new to the human experience. I'm convinced there have been ADHDers ever since our earliest ancestors climbed down from the trees. Do I have a time machine with which to verify this theory? Sadly, no. And I'm not a genetic anthropologist, so I don't have expertise in the science tools that could check this theory in non–time travel ways. I'm just a guy with a hunch.

But I think it's a pretty good hunch.

Regardless of my hunch, the main point here is that humans have been using strategies to deal with ADHD symptoms since long before modern chemistry brought us stimulant medications. The real thing that's changed about the human experience in the last couple hundred years is that we're more compartmentalized, industrialized, and citified than we've been throughout most of history. A lot of things about being a biological human were easier to keep in balance before the invention of things like elevators and smartphones.

So, in this section, we'll focus on general mind and body maintenance stuff.

Here's the basic bullet points for the first chunk:

- exercise and activity
- eating healthy
- healthy sleep habits

- meditation
- connection and community

I know. These are the things they tell everybody to work on. But guess what? ADHDers technically qualify as belonging to the all-inclusive concept of everybody. There is no “exemption from taking care of the body” clause in the ADHD contract.

[h2]Do I really have to exercise?

Yeah. It’s a really great idea to get regular exercise. Our brains were designed to operate in bodies that move. If you don’t keep the body moving, all the systems get out of whack. For ADHDers, because our inborn mechanisms for dopamine and norepinephrine release are already glitchy, when we aren’t active, our levels of those key neurotransmitters go into the toilet.

It’s not a coincidence that adult ADHD diagnosis rates went up when COVID shutdowns encouraged everyone to stay on the couch for a year.

Moving the body, elevating the heart rate, and getting out and about all do wonders for the brain. Exercise that gets the heart rate up specifically releases a protein called the brain-derived neurotrophic factor (BDNF). This protein bolsters the nerve cells operating while you exercise. And there are a lot of nerve cells operating when you exercise. BDNF even encourages the growth of new neurons and brain connections. This heightened connectivity boosts the release of norepinephrine and dopamine.

Study after study shows brain activity, concentration, and attention—all of it—benefit after twenty minutes of exercise.

Also there’s the benefits of maintaining strength and cardiovascular function and all that other good stuff that will help extend that statistically shortened lifespan of the average ADHDer.

What if I’m not able to exercise?

I hear you. What you’re saying is real. I’m not trying to exercise-shame anyone. Because, you know, shame doesn't get anyone anywhere helpful.

Not everyone is able to exercise at the level that the word *exercise* implies. Some people have mobility issues. Other people have conditions that cause chronic pain, or even some complications from long COVID that counterintuitively cause inflammation or other issues that can lead to a net negative effect from exercise. Sometimes we have some built-up emotional blocks from pushing ourselves too hard and getting hurt every time we've tried exercise. Those emotional blocks are no small deal. In the moments when those emotional blocks kick in, they can be as paralyzing as a physical injury. (These emotional blocks can be similar to, or happen concurrently with, a related shame response/rejection crash/RSD moment.)

There are a whole lot of valid reasons why activity may be limited for a person. I don't want to tell anyone to do anything that they can't actually do. That would be a dick move.

At the same time, I want to encourage everybody to be active at a level that is right for them. Don't overdo it. But try being mindful about what happens with your brain when you do anything active. Is there a sweet spot that helps your mental well-being without hurting your physical well-being?

It could be that there just isn't a sweet spot. Or there is a sweet spot, but it requires a physical therapist or family member to help you do it.

At the very least, there can be a benefit from just moving to a different chair and getting a different view for a while. Get outside. If you can touch grass, touch grass. Remember to honor what activity you do get in, even if it doesn't seem like exercise. Give yourself credit for doing it. Recognizing the accomplishment can give you a dopamine boost in itself.

If you absolutely can't go there with exercise and activity, that's cool. Hopefully another strategy can be helpful.

What if I can't stand the thought of going to a gym?

Don't go to a gym, then. Build in some activity elsewhere. Go for a walk. Ride a bike. Do yoga. Go up and down the stairs a couple times for no reason. Play with your kids.

For years, bike commuting was part of my activity routine. It was great. I always felt better at work when I rode my bike. I didn't feel the need to stress eat all day. I could roll with setbacks and changes in plans. It was great!

Then a big construction project happened on the main route from my home to my job. There were plenty of workarounds, but all the same, that disruption was enough to knock me out of the habit. This is just to say, while activity is great, be vigilant about disruptions to your routine. Keep it varied. Keep it interesting.

How do I get motivated to exercise?

The best motivation is recognizing the benefit you get when you exercise. Pay attention to how you feel as the BDNF works its magic (and by magic, I mean science) on your nervous system. Remembering that immediate neurochemical reward you get while exercising is a much more powerful motivator than feeling guilty about how you missed leg day because a work meeting creeped up on you.

Some people benefit from having a set routine with scheduled workout times. When the phone alert for "time to exercise" goes off, they stop what they're doing and go to the gym. Or they run up and down the stairs. Or do yoga. Whatever it is, they do it.

It takes a certain kind of simple brain discipline to follow that schedule reminder. The weird truth is, the less time you spend thinking about whether you want to listen to the reminder, the more effective it is. It can work, but only if you don't think about it. Just jump up and go to the gym, or whatever.

No need to give me the long list of why having such a routine couldn't possibly work for you. I have a similar collection of partially-used day planners and abandoned schemes.

Side Quest:

Tai Chi

Recently, between drafts of this book, I started doing tai chi. I found a really basic tai chi for beginners video on YouTube and gave it a shot. Almost immediately, I noticed I was having a much better time with emotional regulation. Seriously. A seven-minute routine of gentle movements and balance exercises helped me not lose my shit on a daily basis.

And why it works should have been so painfully obvious to me long ago, but it's hard to build new habits, right? Basically, it's an easy movement routine that I can do anywhere, that engages opposite sides of the body, and that makes me practice my balance. I know intellectually that doing all those things engages my brain in a way that helps my brain work better. It just took me a while to get off my butt and try it.

I still need to figure out how to work some cardio into my day, though. Tai chi is definitely not cardio.

That's why I come back to the trick of remembering the neurochemical reward of exercise. Just think about that boost of good feels you got from that last twenty-minute session on the stationary bike. It'll make you feel like you want to get on the bike for twenty minutes.

How hard should I exercise?

Short answer, hard enough to get your heart rate up for a while without hurting yourself. "No pain, no gain" is self-destructive bullshit. How are you going to remember how good that burst of neurochemicals feels when your pain receptors are screaming at you?

Sure, going to the threshold of pain in your workout is how you grow muscle mass. But your workout doesn't have to be about bodybuilding. If that's what you're going for, totally. Do some research. Consult a personal trainer. But, for the mission of improving your ADHD brainspace, you don't need to be that hardcore. You're just aiming for the basic maintenance level of activity that supports good mental health.

If you have been in the habit of quarantine-era levels of inactivity, ease into it. Don't jump off the couch thinking you can run a marathon. Start out with some stretching. If something starts hurting, take care of it. Try to keep the impulsivity urge from making you push it too hard. You have plenty of time to work up to an activity and exercise program.

What if I fall out of the exercise habit?

Don't beat yourself up about it. Things happen in life that throw off our routines. It's normal. Give yourself grace. Try not to feed into the kind of shame spiral that makes it harder and harder to get back on the yoga ball. You aren't a failure because work got really busy for a few weeks and you literally had to choose between sleep or exercise.

Remember how good the exercise-induced neurochemical boost

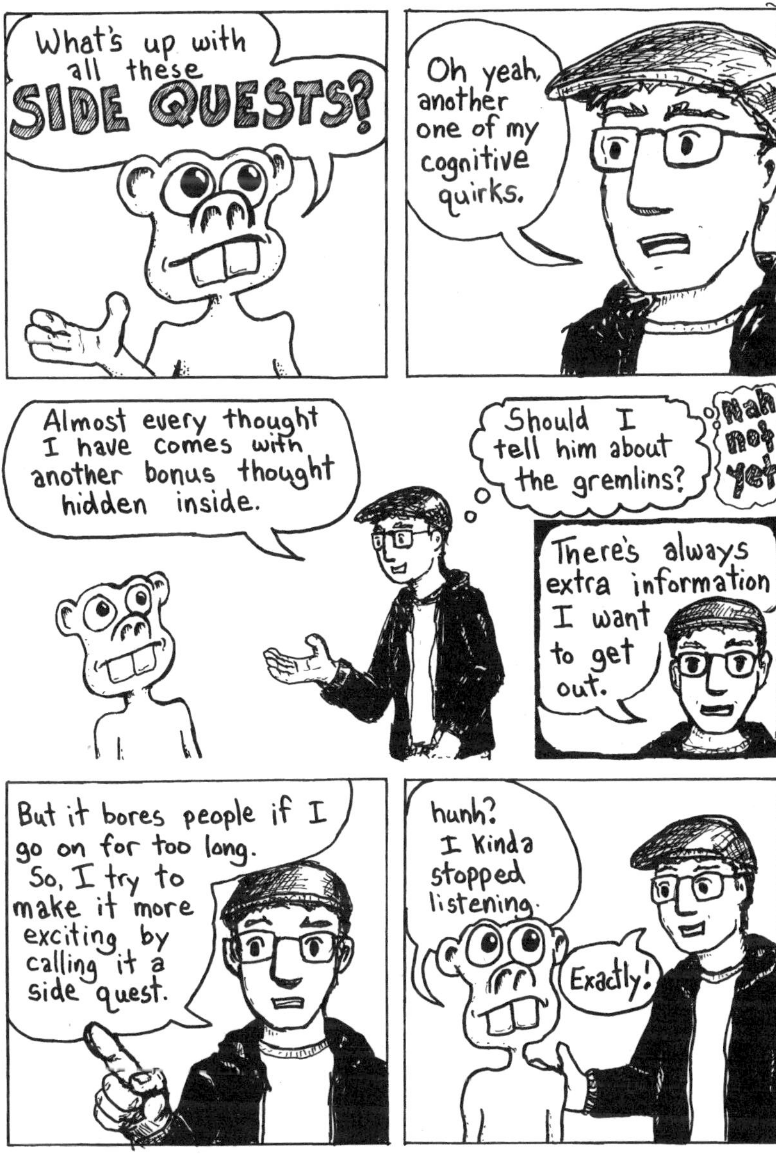
What's up with all these SIDE QUESTS?
Oh yeah, another one of my cognitive quirks.
Almost every thought I have comes with another bonus thought hidden inside.
Should I tell him about the gremlins?
Nah not yet
There's always extra information I want to get out.
But it bores people if I go on for too long. So, I try to make it more exciting by calling it a side quest.
hunh? I kinda stopped listening.
Exactly!

feels and do a few wall push-ups. You eased yourself into the exercise habit before, you can ease yourself back in, now. I believe in you.

When you say "eating healthy," how healthy are we talking?

We're talking about balance. Making sure you get some fresh fruits and vegetables. Remembering to eat at regular times. Being mindful about how much sugar and fried foods you're putting into your body.

No need to worry about going keto or vegan, or whatever. (Unless you want to go on that journey. In which case, best of luck to you. You'll have to consult someone else's book for the details, though.)

In essence, what I mean by "healthy eating" is getting into the habit of considering how the foods you eat are going to affect how your body works. What foods are going to make you feel good throughout the day? How often do you need to eat in order to maintain an even energy level? What foods are going to spike your energy in a sudden and publicly embarrassing way? What foods cause inflammation? What foods are going to send you to the toilet in a sudden and possibly publicly embarrassing way?

I know. That's a hard ask in America, where the prevailing cultural paradigm begs you to continually shovel comfort bites into your food hole all the waking hours.

Do I really need to give up my steady stream of comfort bites?

Of course not. It would be unethical of me to tell you to give up something I can't shake myself. I can only encourage you to be mindful about what it is you put in your mouth when you have that need to munch on something.

Does it have to be cookies? (I am *so* good at mindlessly shoving cookies into my mouth). Or could it be some apple slices? And does the thought of cutting up an apple make you realize you're not actually hungry? Do you really just need an excuse to walk around for a bit?

The answers to these questions will vary depending on what you realize your body actually needs. The point isn't to talk yourself out of eating half a family size package of Oreos. It's to slow down the impulse and to see what it's really responding to.

What is that stress eating impulse about?

Unfortunately, mindless stress eating actually addresses a couple common problems ADHDers face. It's a maladaptive strategy, for sure. But in the land of pre-packaged carbs and fats, it's a really easy strategy to implement.

One of the problems stress eating tackles is that it quickly delivers reward stimulus to a brain that is desperate for it. For an ADHDer, a lot of the tasks required by modern adult life are just so unstimulating and unpleasant. Sitting at a workstation for hours. Reading emails, writing emails, wondering why the fuck people write so many emails, seriously wondering why people send inane reply-all responses to all-staff emails. There are other painfully unstimulating adult tasks, like folding laundry or organizing the doom piles. The point is, the weight of this mind-numbing minutia leaves the ADHD brain craving some different input.

Eating something, especially if it has some simple carbohydrates that quickly convert to glucose, triggers a dopamine release. And, as discussed earlier, dopamine is one of the key neurotransmitters that the ADHD brain has trouble keeping in circulation. The brain is instantly getting rewarded by that dopamine boost and we can get right back to work.

Unfortunately, the sugar rush burns off pretty quickly. It's not a sustained boost. Other mechanisms in the body, developed during our hunter-gatherer past, get to work converting the extra glucose into fat to be stored until some unforeseen future crisis requires it.

But the ADHDer's boredom crisis isn't in the future, it's right now, so another cookie or soda or donut is in order. And don't even try to fool yourself into thinking diet soda will do the trick. You'll get the sweetness, sure, but you won't get the glucose-induced dopamine release. So you end up stress eating other carbs to make up for the lack of reward from your aspartame fizzy drink.

So what's the stress eater to do? Eat some fruits and vegetables instead of grabbing the baked goods. Seriously. Don't worry about the glycemic index of those carrot sticks, or whatever it is the low-carb diet people say. The sugars bound up in whole fruits and vegetables take more time for the body to process than the highly refined stuff in the pre-packaged cookies. You'll get that snack-related dopamine boost, but it'll come in a more even and sustained way.

Why do ADHDers have trouble making healthy meals?

Food prep is a struggle for some of us. It can demand a lot out of our executive function, our working memory, and our sense of object permanence. These are three key areas of weakness for ADHDers.

You know how one of the classic ADHD symptoms is time-blindness? I'm pretty sure I suffer from "refrigerator blindness." It is super difficult for me to figure out what is going on in a refrigerator. Especially if it is a refrigerator I share with someone else. It's as though the simple act of opening the refrigerator door clears out my working memory cache and suddenly I am hunter-gatherer Ogg trying to find what's edible in the primeval boreal forest.

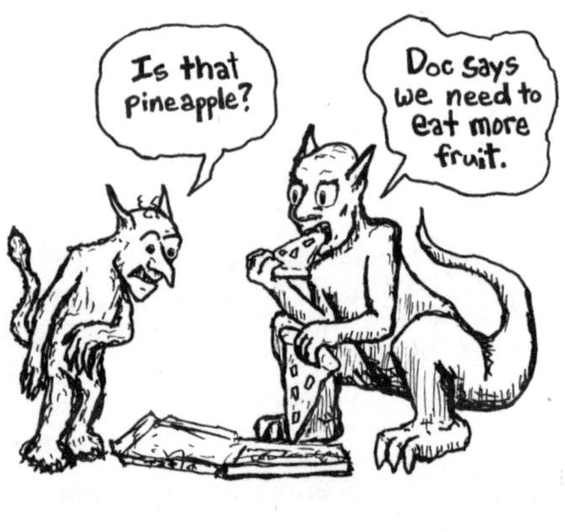
Is that pineapple?
Doc says we need to eat more fruit.

I have been very lucky to have spent the last nine years sharing a refrigerator with a foodie who likes to cook. It's been wonderful. But every once in a while, my partner will be out of town or to dinner with friends. Then, it's just me and the fridge. There are three or four things I routinely reach for. I know where they are. I put them in the fridge myself. One of those things is beer. The other is the milk I pour on the cereal I have for breakfast everyday. And I can usually find the cheese.

The rest of that stuff? I have no idea what it is or what it's for. Maybe it's part of a recipe my partner's going to make later in the week. Is it safe to eat some of it, or will I screw up the whole system? And then there's a big container of plain yogurt. I don't know what that's about. I only like tiny containers of yogurt with the fruit already in it. That's a one-step snack right there. But we don't have that because, if I bought some, I'd probably forget about it till it expired.

One of the problems is that, when the refrigerator door is closed, it's like everything in there ceases to exist for me. When I open it up, I am struck with the enormity of a flood of brand new information I have to process. I have to either do an in-depth inventory of the fridge's contents in order to understand it, or I can continue in ignorance, so long as I can find the beer I put in there.

And when I close the fridge door, that working memory cache clears before I've even had a chance to develop a sense of object permanence for any of the contents that aren't milk, beer, or cheese.

This is just an illustration of how hard it can be to get to what many neurotypicals might consider the first step in any food preparation process: gathering the ingredients. In fact, I think it's fair to say that on some days, opening the fridge counts as the first step, taking the visual inventory is the second step, and grabbing whatever can be eaten right out of the container is step three.

It can be really hard to make healthy eating choices when the ADHD triple threat of executive function, working memory, and object permanence breakdowns conspire against you.

How do we overcome that food prep triple threat?

My answer is both deceptively simple and seemingly impossible. Implement some systems.

Before you start to spiral into a panic attack about that stack of unused notebooks and day planners in your garage, take a couple deep breaths. I'm not talking about buying some miraculous organizational tool that's going to immediately fall into the darkest pit of your iffy sense of object permanence. I'm talking about creating active systems that cut down the amount of decision-making you have to do when you need to eat.

It's not impossible. There are plenty of ADHDers out there who also have diabetes or hypoglycemia or any number of conditions where having dialed-in food systems is literally a matter of life and death. It's totally possible. If it helps, you can try to motivate yourself by thinking of it as a matter of life and death, but on a longer timeline.

It does take some thinking to get your system set up. And it probably needs regular revisiting as you figure out what works for you and what doesn't. This is the most important part of setting up your system: your system has to work *for* you, not *against* you.

With this in mind, I really can't give you the perfect system. (Honestly, as I am going through a big life change right now, my old system has totally fallen apart and I have to build up a new one that works with my current situation.)

With all that in mind, here is what your system should include:

- Aim for a balance of nutrients. Do a little research and reflection to figure out what proportion of macronutrients (carbohydrates, protein, and fat) work for giving you an even supply of energy through the day. There are plenty of websites and books that can spell this idea out in detail. Some of the faddy diet books may strike you as absolute garbage. They may be absolute garbage. But, also, in my experience, I have found that the advice I have a knee-jerk reaction to often deserves a second pass.

If you're not into doing the deep dive on macros, and I'm right there with you, the basic guiding thought should be to make sure you're not getting all your daily calories from cereal, corn chips, and tater tots. (I have done this. It always seems like a good idea at first, and then, by the end of the day, I feel gross and soggy inside.) The convenience foods of our modern world tip us too far into the carbs and fats territory. Try to balance it out with a fresh vegetable and some lean protein. (Sorry, breaded chicken tenders straight out of the deep fryer do not count as lean.)

- Don't forget about the micronutrients. This is where the fruits and veg come in. Also, taking a daily multivitamin isn't a bad idea. Just make sure you take it towards the end of the day if you use stimulant medications. A big concentrated dose of vitamin C cleanses a lot of things from the system. Amphetamine and methylphenidate drugs are among those things. Best to take the vitamin C at a time when it's not going to work against your medication.
- Find some easy-to-make staple meals. Not every meal has to involve a complicated menu. At some point,I figured out how to make a mean, punk-rock tofu stir-fry. After twenty years of practice, I can do it in twenty minutes, practically blindfolded. (It does help if my partner lets me know which veggies to look for in the fridge, because the fridge blindness is still real.) Think of things you can put together in three or four ingredients that will get you through to the next mealtime. A PB&J and a banana totally counts, and is a much better choice than a handful of chocolate chips. (I know from personal experience that if I eat a handful of chocolate chips instead of lunch, I will

just keep going back to the bag for another handful every few minutes until the bag is empty. I almost never feel the need to make a second PB&J.)

- Eat at regular intervals. Have scheduled meal times. Just like stress eating can be a common ADHD problem, so can forgetting to eat. And they aren't mutually exclusive. I tend to stress eat at work and forget to eat on the weekends. Often, if I am in the hyperfocus flow of a project on which I am my own boss, I will power through for hours until suddenly, I am beset by the shakes. At which point, it is very difficult for me to do any kind of food prep, let alone the healthy kind. If you need to, set alarms on your phone to remind yourself it's time to eat.
- Do some consolidated food prep one day a week. Chop the hell out of veggies. Make some soup or a casserole for several days worth of leftovers.
- Sign up for one of those meal kit services. It's a little pricey, but less expensive than a steady stream of emergency DoorDash orders.
- Have healthy snack foods on hand. I know, the bag of mini sweet peppers costs more than the sale price on the family-size package of cookies, but they'll go farther. Be honest with yourself. Are those cookies going to last more than a day or two in your pantry? The mini peppers—or other conveniently sized, ready-to-eat vegetables—are going to leave you feeling all right on one pass. Add hummus and bread or crackers, and you could even call it a meal.
- Remember that food is fuel and junk food is junk fuel. While the unhealthy options are often cheaper at the outset, fruits and vegetables, lean meats, and whole grains are going to be a more effective fueling option.

Junk food can become a bad habit for anyone. But ADHDers especially need to be on guard because of how vulnerable they are to junk foods' deceptively easy stimulation and dopamine rush.

How can ADHDers develop healthy sleep habits?

Does it help you to know it's 3:30 AM as I write this? There is no reason I am awake other than that my brain started spinning an hour ago. So I figured I'd better get up and do something with that energy.

The ADHDer's struggle with getting rest is real. The goal isn't to hit 100% perfect sleep. The goal is to do the best you can with a brain that likes to switch gears without warning.

Sometimes that means going from a dead sleep to suddenly waking up with a new and perfect idea for a project or problem that's been on the mental back burner for months.

Other times, the quality of dead sleep was never part of the equation. The looming deadline of bedtime has suddenly provided an imperative to get those tasks done that have been lost to procrastination all day. The hyperfocus has kicked in and along with it, the naive notion that you don't really need as much sleep as normal people anyway. Some people refer to this as "revenge bedtime procrastination." I'm only mentioning the term because some people find it meaningful. I just find it confusing. The autistic part of me has trouble figuring out who is the recipient of this vengeance.

Regardless of who is being revenged upon, the ADHD brain needs rest and recovery as much as anyone else. Maybe even more so. The amount of brain power needed to keep an even keel in the neurotypical-dominant cultural paradigm is exhausting.

So how do you get enough rest?

- Make yourself a sleep routine and try to stick to it. If you have a consistent wake time and bedtime, your body is going to have a better time maintaining the balance of your neurotransmitters.

- Have a regular pre-bedtime routine. The teeth brushing and getting pajamas on and laying out tomorrow's outfit or tools or whatever. Have a pattern of winding-down activities that let your brain know it's sleepytime. If this sounds awfully like how you prepare a small child for bed, it is. Children are people. People actually will follow a predictable pattern most of the time when one is offered to them. The tricky thing about being a grown-up is remembering how much the pattern depends on you, yourself, reinforcing that pattern.
- Put the screens away an hour before sleepytime. Seriously, ADHDers tend to have a higher sensitivity to light, which means the light from your doom-scrolling phone is going to rev up your alertness brain molecules way more than it does for neurotypicals. This alertness trigger from the light of the screens tends to buddy up with time-blindness in a mean way. Don't believe me? Just think about the last time you sat down to watch one episode of a show and ended up binge-watching half a season.
- Don't hit snooze. Get out of bed when that alarm goes off. This reinforces to your body that the wakeful part of the twenty-four hour cycle has started. Getting in enough wakefulness before bedtime will help with that bedtime routine.

But what if I have multiple jobs and/or small children and/or loud neighbors and/or midnight basketball that make it impossible to have a regular sleep schedule?

I absolutely understand that there are at least eight billion legitimate reasons why regular sleep is hard to come by. The hope is that these reasons are due to temporary situations and your life will soon fall into a regular pattern. But it may not.

Some people are haunted by a sleeplessness that originates beyond the roots of ADHD. I grew up with a combat veteran in the house. Undiagnosed PTSD was part of the ambient environment. My dad leaned into his sleeplessness in a major way, taking every extra shift his railroad job offered. This meant the whole house operated in a weird twilight world, timing our lives around my dad who, when he was home, was either on the edge of exhaustion, or trying real hard to catch up on everything he missed.

Which is to say, I did not have good sleep habits modeled for me. I know that for some of us, sleep comes when we can get it. And, in that case, the trick is to make the most of what we get.

Okay, Mr. Genius, how do I pull off that trick?

The first thing is to learn how not to be furious about the situation. Fury is not conducive to sleep. Being able to accept that you're having trouble getting sleep without compounding the problem with frustration, anger, and howling is some next-level mindfulness shit. It's not easy. And I'm pretty sure the low-dose SSRI I take for anxiety every night before bed helps take some of that edge off.

But I had trouble sleeping long before I got prescribed that med. Like, since forever. And I did create a couple tricks along the way:

- Don't look at clocks when you're trying to sleep. Give yourself the opportunity to let your time-blindness work for you, not against you. Long ago, I decided that if I didn't let myself look at a clock, then time didn't exist. It's a lie, sure. But, there are situations when noting the passage of time isn't really helpful. Those moments when you are hoping to intentionally lose consciousness are not times to look at the clock. Turn the clocks away from your bed if you have to. Or get one of those old-timey analog clocks that don't glow all night long. And keep your phone more than an arm's reach away from your sleeping spot.

- Consider that, while lying quietly with your eyes closed might not be actual sleep, it can be a close second. Especially if you're able to lie there quietly without getting furious about how you're not asleep.
- Try a podcast or an audiobook. Pick one that's really boring or repetitive. There are actually podcasts out there specifically designed to bore people to sleep. It might work for you. There's nothing more likely to help an ADHDer zone out than somebody talking about boring stuff. Back in the days when I had basic cable, I went through a phase where I slept with the Weather Channel playing softly in the background. This strategy might be difficult to employ if you share a sleeping area with someone.
- Learn when your regular highs and lows in energy are during the day. For whatever reason, American culture likes to ignore the biological reality of what human beings' activity cycles are actually like. An individual's natural wakeful periods change over their lifetime. Teenagers actually have a biological bias towards staying up late and sleeping later in the day. Older adults often need less sleep than people in their thirties and forties. People in their twenties try to convince themselves they don't need sleep. There are theories about the social and evolutionary advantages of having these staggered sleep cycles across a multi-generational community. There's also the theory that eight straight hours of overnight sleep is a relatively new development for humans. Our bodies might be better suited to a segmented sleep cycle with a period of wakefulness between a couple three- to five-hour sleep segments. All that to say, your body's natural rhythms might be at odds with the American industrial concept of the 9-to-5 workday. If that schedule really isn't working for

you, explore what changes you can make to accommodate the times you are naturally more prone to rest.

- Caffeine naps are an option. If this sounds absurd, you might be a VASTie and not an ADHDer. But ADHDers tend to have a counterintuitive response to afternoon caffeine. Way before I got the ADHD diagnosis, I enjoyed coming home from work in the afternoon, having whatever coffee was left in the pot, and lying down on the couch for a power nap. Caffeine works on different neurotransmitters than the ADHD meds do. It generally helps with alertness and countering the effects of fatigue. And a lot of ADHDers enjoy those effects most of the time. But there's also something darn relaxing about that coffee in the afternoon.

These tricks might not work for you. Some of them might seem to contradict each other. The brain's an interesting place. Some things work for some situations sometimes. But isn't that a relief? You don't have to be locked into the same sleep routine for the rest of your life. You can switch it up as life circumstances change.

How can meditation help?

You might be asking, "Is this like woo-woo stuff?" Not necessarily. Unless you like woo-woo stuff. Because anything that adds excitement and flavor to an activity staves off boredom, the universal enemy to ADHDers. If you want your meditation practice to include special effects, costumes, and fancy candles, don't let me stop you.

But that's a lot of stuff to keep track of.

Is there a non-woo-woo way to meditate?

There are many. The easiest is to just focus on your breathing. Keep track of that in and out pattern. Try to let go of any extraneous thoughts and focus on being a body that breathes for a couple minutes. There are a lot of different breathing patterns you can try.

Square breathing is a simple one: breathe in for a count of four; hold for a count of four; breathe out for a count of four; hold for a count of four; then repeat the pattern a few times.

Are there ways to meditate that don't involve sitting absolutely still and quiet?

You bet! There's a thing called walking meditation, which is really just going for a walk. The rhythm of your body low-key works some of the meditation magic on your brain without you having to think about not thinking. Running or biking can help the same way.

And there are some even more focused and sustained active meditation practices. Yoga is a great twofer. It also builds in balance activities that stimulate the cerebellum. If yoga's not active enough, you can try martial arts—where the precision movements actually help the brain's overall focus.

So you're saying I could become a ninja to treat my ADHD?

I'm not saying you couldn't, but that sounds like a stretch.

Connection and community? In this day and age?

I know we're all damaged goods traveling through a hyper-commodified landscape full of opportunistic zombies looking to devour our precious brains and consume our free will.

But are we? Really?

Or does it just feel like that because we're isolating ourselves to guard against future damage from the neurotypical-dominant cultural paradigm?

ADHDers often have a lot of baggage around previous social exchanges. Many ADHDers had childhoods where they felt disproportionately blamed for every problem that arose. Like, sure, some of the stuff may have been their fault, but a lot of times, they'd get blamed for something that happened on the other side of the classroom. Or worse. Neurotypical kids have a knack for knowing who to deflect blame to when being questioned by the vice principal. They figure that the impulsive kid who's always in trouble makes the perfect patsy to catch the heat for their own calculated mischief. And that's just the damage from fourth through eighth grade. And these are the tamer examples. A lot of people go through much worse, and I'm not trying to make light of their experiences.

So, it absolutely makes sense that ADHDers have a lot of skepticism when it comes to trusting other people. At the same time, ADHDers have a lot of optimism when it comes to trusting other people. It's another one of the many paradoxes in this condition of contradictions.

That optimism comes from the excitement of interacting with people. Other people are surprising and unpredictable. There is often something new to learn from them. They might invite you to join them on adventures. Conversations can be exciting and rev up a lot of those precious neurotransmitters. Especially if there's flirting involved!

But then there's the confusion, the disappointment, and the debilitating rejection crash (or rejection-sensitive dysphoria, as some people like to call it), when a misunderstanding or disagreement arises. And of course, this rejection crash is often informed by a history of disappointment, rejection, and confusion.

So, when I say connection and community are important, I know that makes some people want to throw a chair at me.

It's fine. I'm in a different room.

When you're ready, let's dive in.

Why is it important for ADHDers to have positive connections with other people?

Because ADHDers are human beings, and despite how hard the post-modern industrial machine has tried to condition us into living compartmentalized lives in our own private Idahos, human beings need to have regular contact with others. If there's nothing else we learned from the COVID times, it's that people will literally risk their lives breaking lockdown rules because they *need* to go to a party.

Edward M. Hallowell, MD, and John J. Ratey, MD, devoted a whole chapter to "the healing power of connection" in their 2021 book *ADHD 2.0.* I have gone to the well of Hallowell and Ratey so many times in my research, not just because they have those fancy medical doctor credentials, but because they have the ADHD cred too. They are practicing psychiatrists who have been helping out ADHDers, including themselves, for decades. Hallowell and Ratey not only tout the power of "Vitamin Connect," they do so from an ADHDer-lived-experience perspective. They have seen the benefits in themselves, and in their patients, from doing the work of cultivating meaningful relationships and community.

Collaborative and cooperative interactions with other humans make us able to accomplish far more than we could ever do on our own. Having positive and healthy connections to other people can nourish our minds and spirits. (Feel free to interpret the word *spirit* as secularly or religiously as fits your specific comfort level.) Those connections also help us actively participate in the world and keep the body running smoothly. And consensual hugs are great for getting an oxytocin boost.

Do the connections I make online count?

They can. As an old school 90s-era zinester, I can tell you that some very important and meaningful connections are with people I've either never met in person, or only met after years of correspondence and trading zines. So, connections don't have to be made in person. Of course, the online world is its own mess and fraught with dangers. But there are also amazing opportunities to meet people with similar interests who happen to live very far away.

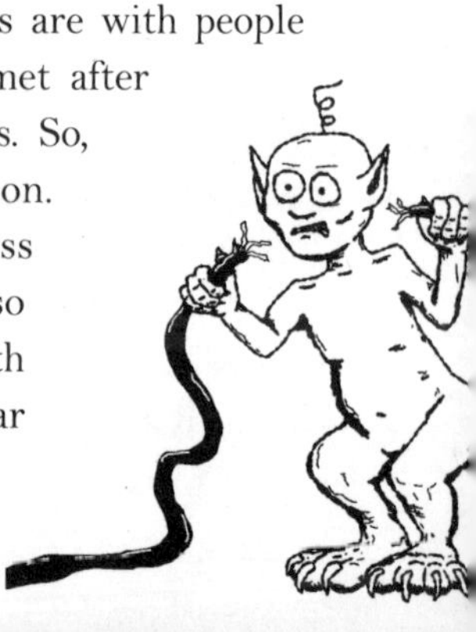

Side Quest:

Oxytocin

Oxytocin is another amazing brain molecule, or neuropeptide, if you want to have the more sciency term. Oxytocin is often called the "love hormone." It gets released during expressions of physical affection, sexual activity, childbirth, and breastfeeding. It is a big deal in the life cycle of a mammalian organism. Oxytocin, along with helping the uterus contract and triggering milk letdown, promotes feelings of security, reduces anxiety, encourages social bonding and trust with the people close to you, and helps out with mood. It even seems to have an effect on wound healing. (Mommy's kiss on a booboo actually does help make it all better.)

One little caveat from the autistic part of my brain: it's possibly good to be very picky about who you hug. If you are easily confused by nonverbal social cues, a hug can be a landmine. The fear of accidentally developing trust with an untrustworthy person is not to be ignored. Consensual hugs from safe people you already know are the best bet.

Some of those old zinester friends made the leap across the digital divide, and we're still connected. These connections count.

During the big COVID shutdown, I started playing an online strategy game. Within the context of the game, I made connections with people and had game-level friendships that were very helpful during the strange, isolating, work-from-home times.

These were low-level connections. And I specifically sought out a game alliance with an international set of players. Partly to practice foreign languages, but also to make sure there was a built-in guardrail to keep from getting too caught up in these people I only knew from an online game context. That guardrail worked for me. After a while, my interest level in the game tapered off (down from a peak of four- to six-hours a day . . . thanks, COVID), and I was able to put it down without feeling like I was letting down my in-game comrades.

Whether online, or in real life, it's important to have some clearly defined boundaries in how you relate to someone. Not every relationship requires the engrossing intensity of a best friend or romantic interest to get the benefits of human connection.

How do I have boundaries while still making connections?

This is not easy. I'm tempted to dodge the whole question and suggest you read Dr. Faith's book *Unfuck Your Boundaries.* Because if you have trouble with personal boundaries, you're going to find a lot of useful information there. If you don't want to go and read that book because you're reading this book, here's my take.

There is a tendency for ADHDers to go all-in on the person who is interacting with them right now, and losing track of the other people in their lives. This can manifest itself in a variety of ways. Maybe it's forgetting to pick up dinner for your family on the way home from work because you got in a really engrossing conversation with a coworker. Maybe it's forgetting how your sexual partner feels about sharing you with other people when that engrossing conversation turns into a couple of drinks and a makeout session in the parking lot.

The important thing to remember is that the boundaries are not just for other people. They're for yourself.

First, think about the circles of connection around you. You're at the center. Depending on how you define such things, your life partner might be right there in the center with you, or in a very tight circle close to the center.[7] Your beloved family members[8] and closest friends might be in the next circle. The next circle out might be your higher interaction friends. You hang out with them or ping them on the internet a lot. The next circle out is your situational contacts. These are your work buddies, fellow special interest club members, business contacts, and friends of friends: you don't often interact with these folx without a situational structure around it. Next out, you've got acquaintances. These are people you know, who know you. You cross paths enough, you generally get along, and they have the potential to move to a closer circle as you get to know more about each other.

And then there's everybody else.

So, with an awareness of which circle of connection another person is in, you can make better decisions about what sorts of actions or activities to do with them. The more you know about a person, the more confidence you can have in moving them to a closer circle. Or not.

For example, I once went with friends/work friends to the Meet Rack, the legendary Tucson dive bar, and was invited by the bartender and a couple day-drunk patrons to join them on the bar's upcoming river rafting trip. Hard pass. I did not know those people. They were in the "everybody else" circle. I would not be

7 It may be that who you think of as your partner doesn't seem to fit so close to you, and you feel they really belong in the closest friends circle. No judgment here. Been there, done that. You get to define your own connection circles.

8 Note the term: "beloved family members." Estranged, frustrating, or unhelpful family members don't need to be in this circle.

engaging in any maritime activities with these people. The only bits of information I had about them was that they were the kind of people who liked day drinking and inviting total strangers on rafting trips. I did not have confidence that I would not be called upon to save them from drowning for doing something stupid. I really didn't want one of these people feeling like they owed me a Wookie-style life debt. They were "everybody else," as far as I was concerned, and they were going to stay "everybody else." So I set a very easily enforceable boundary for myself. I never went to that bar again. (To be fair, the Meet Rack had a reputation for being the kind of bar where you could easily meet people with very low thresholds to their personal boundaries. It really wasn't my kind of place, but I had to at least see what it looked like.)

Most situations are less dramatic. Like, you can take what you know about a person and what circle of connection they're in, to decide how much time or energy you feel okay investing in them. Ideally, the people that give you an equitable return on your time and energy investment are the ones you move to closer connection circles. And that return on energy might come from the simple fact that you enjoy spending time with them. Or it may be that you find you are much more productive in your work or home life because of the interactions you have with that person.

The connection circles are, in a way, a shorthand for the kinds of boundaries you set for different people.

An acquaintance might hit you up for a ride to the airport. But if it's a totally inconvenient time for you, you can easily say no, with no hard feelings expected. If they do give you hard feelings, maybe it's time to shift that acquaintance to "everybody else" land. On the other hand, if you're up for the adventure, giving them the ride might turn out to be the opportunity to have the conversation that moves them up a circle.

A frustrating family member might be hitting you up for a loan or a place to crash one too many times, and you need to kick them to a farther circle. This is harder, but may be necessary.

The thing is to know yourself, what you have to give, what you want to give, and what you're able to give to another person. Also, it's good to keep an eye on what you expect out of other people. If what you're willing to give and what you expect from a person aren't matching up, you probably need to adjust your boundaries.

How do I make sure I don't get into a situation where someone is taking advantage of me?

First off, always have an exit strategy. Before you get too wrapped up in someone, make sure you can get yourself to safety if you need to.

Do you want to drive one hundred miles to the river with the randos from the bar? Are they driving? Are you? Can you get yourself back to civilization when things go south?

There are far worse questions to ask yourself than these, and if you're asking those, it may be time to leave. Sure, the sheer terror of not knowing how the situation will play out may be adding to your feelings of urgency, goosing your norepinephrine levels, and ringing a lot of those ADHD stimulation bells. But is it worth it?

You're not going to get there if you have an exit strategy in mind. Hopefully. There's a lot of tough situations out there that are truly outside our control.

Second thing, try and make sure there's a witness present. Get a buddy to go with you to that first meeting of the LEGO master builders club. Or, if you're out on your own, and someone approaches you with a situation that might be inequitable (usually sales people), create a buddy who's at a different location. Say you've got to check with your partner, go feed your dog, or talk to your parole officer. Whatever will get you out of their circle and on your way.

The third thing is to be very aware of how the things you do—and by *do*, I am including things you ingest—affect your ability to hold your boundaries. Whether it's alcohol or drugs or sex (or fervent denial of sex) or ecstatic religion or, heck, sports fandom, there are a lot of different things people do that will rev up certain neurotransmitters, dial back others, and create feelings of trust towards people we don't actually know that well. Everything is fun and cool, until, all of the sudden, Marshall Applewhite is telling us it's time to free our energy bodies so they can board the flying saucer.

I'm not saying you should never have fun or have a drink or go to church. I'm just saying be mindful of how your brain responds in those situations. Make sure you're not getting in deep with people who really don't care about you, your safety, or your agency as a fully realized human being. Make sure you don't give up your power to say no and that you are able to back up that no by getting the fuck out of there, if necessary.

And it's not always a high-stakes situation where you've got to get out. Sometimes your brain is just jumping out of your body and you need some space and alone time to reset. There have been times when I've been in a car with trusted friends, and suddenly, I just couldn't be in the car anymore. At the time, I couldn't really explain why. It didn't matter, though, because these were trusted friends to whom I had disclosed about my neurodivergence and knew I had pretty significant sensory issues sometimes. And I had a pretty solid track record of being able to get myself home on public transportation, so it wasn't a big deal. And it wasn't personal.

How do I make sure I'm not running over someone else's boundaries?

Let's go back to the well of the Harper family wisdom here. Sammuel E. Harper's zine, *How to Not Be a Dick*, really does a great job at spelling it out in easy-to-understand, Gen Z terminology. It's available from Microcosm, and I highly recommend it. Rather than rehash the whole zine, I'll focus on one of its key points: "Treat others the way they want to be treated."

This basically boils down to not assuming other people want

what you want out of an interaction or situation.

Everyone's a little different. When you have ADHD, you are different from the neurotypical majority. Unfortunately, for us ADHDers, this often means needing to do some extra empathy work on our part when we're dealing with neurotypicals. This is where good, honest, and open communication comes in handy. This is especially important for the people you have, or want to have, in your closest circles of connection. Listen to the other person and get to know what's important to them. You'll be surprised how much value you can add to a relationship just by recognizing the things that make them happy and pointing them out when you notice them.

And, by the same token, you can learn what makes them unhappy, annoyed, and pissed off. Some of these things will be the tiniest details you barely even think about. But it's not about you. Not at this point.

Hopefully, as you are doing the empathy work of learning about the other person, they are learning similar things about how you like to be treated. If they aren't, maybe they don't deserve to be in such a close circle of connection. You can let them naturally slip out to a further circle without much effort. You don't even have to be a dick about it.

How can ADHDers get along better with other people?

The main thing you need to know is that 80% of people have trouble accepting that not everyone's brains work like theirs do. There's a lot of stuff about you that they are really not going to understand on the first pass.

You've got two options for helping them understand where your brain is coming from.

1) You can become a super advocate and bust your butt trying to advance the Neurodiversity Movement in all areas of your life.

2) You can give the important people in your life a copy of this book. (Or another ADHD book you like better. There's a bunch of them in the references section at the end of this book.) Tell them it would be really meaningful for you if they read it.

If the first option sounds exhausting, it is. The second option can be a bit daunting as well.

There's always option three, keeping it to yourself and faking normal as best you can. But you've probably already been doing that for years. It's draining in its own way, and it's hard to have solid and meaningful connections with other people if you are always hiding an important part of yourself from them.

Luckily, you don't have to go all-in on any one of these options. In fact, it might be better if you don't. Take it slowly. Figure out who you are, then figure out how to genuinely present yourself to the world around you. Do the personal work of figuring out how to best get your brain to work for you before you start proselytizing the ADHD-Awareness Gospel to the masses.

There are already scads of social media influencers shouting in the algorithmic echo chambers and a lot of them still have a ways to go on their journey. Of course, if making TikToks about ADHD is part of how you do your personal work, well, that sounds messy and public, but you do you.

I strongly advise you to start small and with your closest circles of connection. Cultivate those inner circles judiciously. Seek more connection with the people who value you for who you are, are able to recognize your strengths, and don't have a problem picking up the slack when your weaknesses come into play.

Then, move to the outer circles, the people who don't care to make the effort to understand you. There are plenty of folx in the outer circles of connection who don't really need to know how your brain works, and that's fine. Just try to remember that they are in an outer circle and don't need the same amount of attention from you as your

Side Quest:

Neurodivergent Friends

I'm not sure what kind of sociological studies have actually been done on this, but from plenty of anecdotal evidence, personal experience, and stuff I see on the internet, neurodivergent people tend to clump together. It is not unheard of for an ADHDer and someone of a different neurodivergent type to become best friends. Many of my longtime friends have turned out to have some sort of brain interestingness. Whether it's dyslexia, or bipolar, or autism, or ADHD, or Tourette's, or any of the other many conditions under the neurodivergence umbrella.

I think we just sense when we're around other neurodivergent people and we relax a bit. We feel more comfortable being ourselves. We know they're less likely to get weirded out by our eccentric social quirks. We lose the compulsion to mask so hard when we're around other neurodivergent folx. It's a figurative breath of fresh air.

Long story short, it's pretty frickin' great to have neurodivergent friends.

inner circles. Be patient with them, but don't let them drag you down.

Most importantly, know who you are. Know what you need and build the structure in your life that gives it to you. Remember to celebrate your wins. Try not to dwell any more on your losses than what you need to learn from them. When you've got yourself figured out, all your relationships with other people are going to run much smoother.

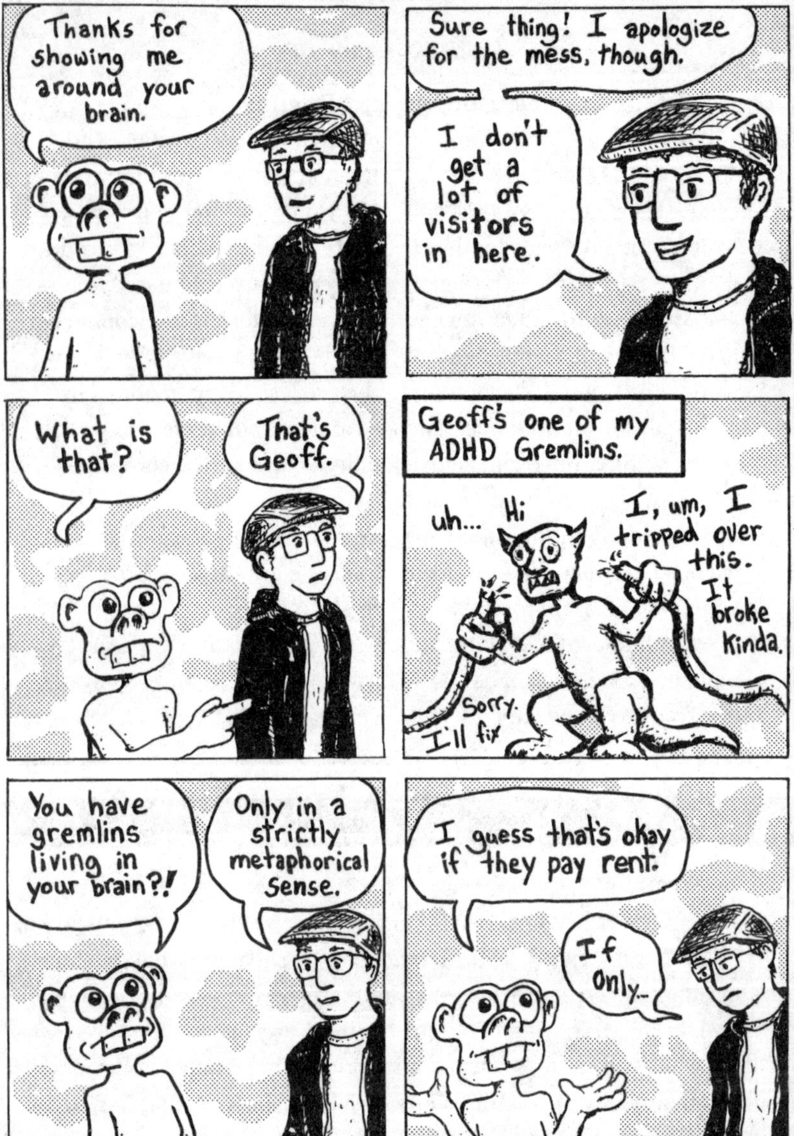
Thanks for showing me around your brain.
Sure thing! I apologize for the mess, though.
I don't get a lot of visitors in here.
What is that?
That's Geoff.
Geoff's one of my ADHD Gremlins.
uh... Hi
I, um, I tripped over this. It broke kinda.
Sorry. I'll fix
You have gremlins living in your brain?!
Only in a strictly metaphorical sense.
I guess that's okay if they pay rent.
If only...

ADHD-SPECIFIC PROBLEMS

The previous section was pretty broad, covering general human being maintenance strategies. Even if they are pretty general, you can use them to maximize your own body's ability to get the brain chemicals where you want them. But, for ADHDers, while basic human maintenance strategies are very useful, they don't cover everything. This section focuses on tips for the specific problems ADHDers encounter.

Where the hell did I put my keys?

Here's a fun fact. If someone else misplaces their keys, I'm really good at finding them quickly. If I misplace my own small-but-important item, it might take hours.

The strategy I use is to have a dedicated spot for my important items. As soon as I get home, my keys and wallet are out of my pocket and into their designated spots. I have been doing this since I was a teenager. Maybe even longer.

When I was a weird, undiagnosed teenager, it really bugged me when I couldn't find these things. If I neglected to put my wallet or keys in their spots, I would almost instantly not be able to find them again. It didn't make any sense to me, either, that these things would just disappear because I set them in a different spot. It was almost as if some supernatural creature out of Jim Henson's *Labyrinth* was moving them around just to mess with me. And then, as I mythologized the circumstances even more fully, I realized that the supernatural creatures could only move my keys and wallet if I *didn't* put them in the keys and wallet spot.

If I was very deliberate in placing things in their specific homes,

I could foil these creatures' mischief. I bought in fully to the idea that pixies were stealing my stuff and hiding it with their magic. It gave me a very simple explanation as to why I couldn't find the damn things even when they were in plain sight. And it gave me a fun and engaging way to think about the problem.

Of course, now I know it's not pixies playing pranks on me: it's ADHD gremlins yanking on the DMN/TPN switches before I can file my objects' locations into short-term memory.

So, right there, I've employed two strategies to keep track of my keys. First, I have created a dedicated spot for them and consistently use it. Second, I heighten the importance of using the designated location by imagining supernatural creatures are going to mess with me if I don't.

What's the strategy for not losing things?

Always put them in the same place and create for yourself a very memorable reason why you need to put the things there.

If need be, you can make it a very exaggerated reason enhanced with thoroughly imagined visualizations. Ridiculous things are easier to remember than boring ones. Make it a little bit gross, and it becomes even more memorable. Like, if you have trouble unpacking after trips, create for yourself a reason you need to get that suitcase emptied and sorted ASAP. That reason may be that at midnight, a family of raccoons will break into your home, rifle through the unpacked bags, and have angry diarrhea on any travel items or passports they see lying out of place.

It's absolutely absurd, but the absurdity will spark your penchant for novelty, which will help you get an otherwise tedious task done.

How do I decide what the right place to put something is?

I'm going to be honest. A room in my house is full of piles of things that are yet to be assigned to a spot. These are lovingly referred to as my "doom piles." Until I can figure out a home for each item in the

Side Quest:

Strategic Object Placement and Motivation

A lot of important items are time-sensitive. Time-sensitive items are doubly hazardous for an ADHDer because they are liable to both the object permanence problem and the time-blindness problem. If the deadline for acting on the time-sensitive item is too far beyond the immediate urgency horizon, the brain doesn't feel it's necessary to do it yet. Which sets us up to procrastinate past the deadline thanks to time-blindness.

However, you can game the system by placing important time-sensitive items in a location that lowers your resistance to acting on them.

For example, when a bill comes in the mail (and for some reason, I still get a couple that way), I put it on my computer keyboard. That way, I am setting it intentionally in a spot where, when I have that automatic need for a distraction from starting other tasks on my computer, I will go to my bank account and schedule the payments. Then I get a little dopamine reward for accomplishing that task, which lowers my resistance to starting the other task I was procrastinating on.

And then, after getting two tasks done, I feel like a freaking superhero and can finally get around to the other thing I've been procrastinating on. If I keep the ball rolling, it is entirely possible I could even get my laundry folded and put away.

pile, it has to stay there. Because when it's in a pile in the middle of my floor, I'm less likely to accidentally forget it exists. Sometimes, an item is moved from a doom pile to on top of my computer keyboard because it's time to do the thing with it, whatever that thing is.

This is a really terrible system, and it makes me nervous. But, it keeps happening, so it must be performing some function, right?

The really remarkable thing is that my piles are, for the most part, contained in this one room. Because there's another side to this coin. I share the house with my wife, who is a very organized person and gets stressed out by visible clutter. She has helped define spots for things in every other room of the house. With the exception of a temporary landing zone on the kitchen island, I have no problem keeping things in their places in all the common areas of our home.

My wife would be more than happy to help me find homes for the things in the doom piles. Especially the cardboard boxes I'm holding onto for mysterious reasons. The only reason I don't let her is because every pile represents a different project I am in process on and will finish, eventually, I promise. I'm worried that if the pile gets sorted I'll forget to ever finish that project.

And here's the function of the doom pile: it's a visual representation and reminder of a project I want to finish.

So, from this scenario we can tease out the simple truth. Having someone help you determine places for things is brilliant. The reason most of the house isn't filled with doom piles is because, as a team, my wife and I figured out was important to each of us in how the house is arranged. So, while there might not be a specific home for everything in the doom piles (yet), my office is actually the perfect temporary home for them while they are in process. Also, there's a door I can close so my wife doesn't have to look at it.

What if I don't have a whole extra room to keep my doom piles in?
Yeah. At one point in my life, when I was moving about every year, the doom piles kept getting churned and purged on a regular basis.

And I was living in tight quarters with someone else in most of those moves.

The constraints of those living situations really limited how much the doom could expand, so it didn't. I'm pretty sure my then-partner would have thrown a bunch of my stuff in the apartment complex dumpster if I didn't keep it in check. We were young and hadn't figured out how to communicate with each other very well and were struggling, in general, with those connection needs human beings have. Of course, it didn't help that I was undiagnosed and unwittingly masking hard all the time. Part of my masking was hiding my piles in cardboard banker's boxes.

It might have been a maladaptive response to a fear that my partner would communicate their displeasure with me by messing with my stuff, but it served a purpose. It is possible to employ a strategy like that in a more proactive way.

There are lots of organizational strategies out there. If you need to have piles, can you keep them in a box and put a lid on it? Does it need to be a transparent box so you can see everything in it? Or would you prefer an opaque box so your doom pile doesn't taunt you in your sleep? Does your system make your life easier? Does it make it easier for the people you live with?

Of course, the simplest strategy is to just designate a zone. If you live in one room of a shared apartment, decide one corner can be your doom zone. If the piles creep out of the zone, take it as a visual signal that you have too much unresolved stuff going on in your life and you need to deal with some of it. Or, get some shelves, so you can expand your doom structure upwards.

Believe it or not, when doom piles are arranged on shelves, they seem less threatening.

How do I deal with time-blindness?

Oh, time-blindness. Some people like to call it "time near-sightedness." Others call it "time optimism." What is the most accurate term? I don't know. I am not a time ophthalmologist, although wouldn't that be cool?

Before I let the default mode network take me down the road of dreaming about the exciting career of time ophthalmology, I'm going to reel it in: there are basically three prongs to this time-blindness business.

First, ADHDers often have an iffy sense of how long it will take to do certain tasks. It's really hard to know when to start a task if you don't have a good sense of how long it will take.

Second, when we get into a flow, we lose track of time passing and find ourselves in a wonderful state of constant now-ness. We are so locked into the TPN because the task, or project, or binge watch at hand provides a constant and steady stream of reinforcing norepinephrine and dopamine.

And the third prong of the time-blindness fork? It has to do with problems keeping track of what's coming up in the future (and the past, sometimes). Like, I might have a good grasp on what's happening today and tomorrow, but next week? How far away is next week? What day is it again? Holy shit! My big deadline is next Tuesday?! (True story. I think today is Thursday. We'll see what happens. If you're reading this book, then it all worked out.)

Like everything else with ADHD, these modes of time-blindness can be a gift or a curse. Or both. The trick is to figure out which guardrails will help you tip the scales toward the gift side.

For the first prong, it is possible to get better at knowing how long tasks will take. Just because your brain does a crappy job remembering how long it takes to do certain tasks doesn't mean you can't use tools outside of your brain to help you.

For example: Every night when my brain is tired, I'm pretty sure it's going to take me at least half an hour to do my bedtime routine. But, I also know that the main reason I had to get an expensive root canal and crown on my left lower incisor is that I skipped nighttime flossing for five years. (And skipped going to the dentist, but for different reasons.) But the truth is, my routine actually just takes me five minutes. Pajamas, nighttime meds and vitamins, floss, two minutes with the sonic toothbrush, and a couple seconds to put on the goop that keeps the toenail fungus at bay.

Knowing from experience that it will only take five minutes helps me. Especially since it's such a practiced routine I can slip right into DMN and muscle memory takes care of the rest.

There are a lot of simple, everyday tasks that ADHDers will avoid because it feels like it will take way too much time, and the couch is calling. Or, we know there is something really important we have to do at 5:00 PM and we don't want to accidentally slip into that second prong of time-blindness. We know it is entirely possible, from experience, to get into the flow on a project, and forget all about the really important thing on the schedule. So, maybe it's safer, if less productive, to stay on the couch and do nothing but mentally prepare and obsess over the 5:00 PM appointment. I'm not saying this is a good strategy. I'm just saying this is what a lot of us do if we don't have strategies in place.

What are the strategies I can use to help with time-blindness?

- Try data collection. Use a stopwatch to see how long it actually takes to do some basic tasks. Write these times down somewhere useful to you. Maybe it's an old-fashioned paper notebook. Maybe it's a whiteboard you keep somewhere very visible. Maybe it's an app on your phone. The point is, don't burden your brain with the task of keeping track of that information. Write that stuff down somewhere it's easy to refer to.

- Analyze the data. Use the data you've collected to decide which tasks to do and how many of them you can accomplish during a certain amount of clock time.

- Utilize biologically built-in rewards. Remind yourself that completing tasks will give you a dopamine boost. Imagine how good it will feel to have that laundry folded and put away. (I'm trying to imagine it myself right now.) If you can get started on a task that you know is doable in a documented amount of time, you know you can get that dopamine kick at the end of that time interval. Use that knowledge to light a fire under your ass and get some of those little things done while you're killing time before the big thing at 5:00.
- Try timers and alarms. I often use the basic timer on my phone to remind me to move on to the next task. So use your time-keeping technology to give structure to your day. I was already using this tool when the therapist I first talked to about ADHD recommended dialing it up. He specifically said not to regard that alarm as an option. When the reminder to go to the gym pops up, go to the gym. (I have yet to set that particular reminder, but you get the idea.)
- Utilize data-based urgency manipulation: If you have something important to do at a certain time in the afternoon, set an alarm for yourself for the time you need to start the process of getting to it. Don't set the alarm for when you're supposed to be there. Use the data you've collected to work backwards and determine what time you need to get off the couch and get together whatever you need to be able to arrive on time. Then, when that alarm goes off, allow the sense of urgency to flood your brain with norepinephrine. You will keep on track because not only do you have the data on what you need to do, and how long you need to do it, you have an adrenal hormone helping you out.

- Employ a white board/vision board/cork board/kitchen graffiti: For those things that are coming up, but are over your immediate time horizon, make some kind of visual system of marking them. Believe it or not, doom piles are a very rudimentary form of this kind of visual reminder system. But you don't have to trip over the piles. Have a visible list on a wall of things that are coming up. Try to put them in order so that it's clear which is the soonest. White boards are pretty handy for this kind of thing. But, if you hate white boards because they remind you of school or work, use something else that serves the same function. The important thing is that upcoming things are visible and marked with a date when they will occur. And remember to remove expired items from the board.

How can I get past ADHD paralysis/stalled executive function?

So, first of all, ADHD Paralysis or "analysis paralysis," or any other buzzwordy way of putting it, is not to be confused with neuromuscular paralysis, which is a very frightening, very real condition. In fact, any kind of physically disabling paralysis of a permanent or long-term nature is a whole deal not to be taken lightly. When ADHDers say they are experiencing ADHD paralysis, they are pretty much talking about having trouble getting their executive function in gear. It's often a temporary, transitory thing—unlike a severe spinal injury or a muscle-wasting disease, or any of the other major medical reasons we probably shouldn't be throwing around the word *paralysis* so lightly. No offense to anyone who likes the other phrase, but I'm going to suggest we call this particular ADHD experience "stalled executive function."

Okay, fine, how do I get past stalled executive function?

When you can't get out of bed or off the couch to do any of the

Side Quest:

The Famous Tomato Timer Technique

When Italian business guy Francesco Cirillo[1] was an undergraduate student, he just could not pay attention to his sociology textbook. He kept getting distracted. But he figured out an external support to keep himself going. He happened to have a kitchen timer that was in the shape of a tomato. He challenged himself to focus on the textbook for twenty-five minutes, then have a five-minute break before doing another rep. It worked for him, and he figured it might work for other people. He also figured if he trademarked the Italian word for tomato, *pomodoro*, he could sell a lot of tomato-shaped timers to people who wanted to learn his productivity management technique. His personal biography doesn't say anything about ADHD, but this method can work for maintaining focus on less appealing tasks. It does require a rigorous adherence to the authority of the timer, which I've never been able to manage for more than two repetitions. But, why not try it? 25 minutes on task, 5 minutes free time, repeat for four cycles. Two hours of your life has passed and maybe you got something boring done.

1 Francesco Cirillo, "About Francesco - Francesco Cirillo," January 14, 2025, https://www.francescocirillo.com/about.

things swirling around in your brain, that's when your executive function has stalled out. It's like you just can't get the TPN into gear because the DMN won't let you settle on a task to start. (Thanks, ADHD gremlins!)

To get your TPN in gear, use some of the tools we've already talked about. Set a timer for twenty minutes. Tell yourself, "My brain can hang out in the default mode network for twenty minutes, and then I gotta get up." When the timer goes off, get up. Pick one of those tasks and start it. If you can't pick a task, do some jumping jacks or wall push-ups. Run around the block, or just around the inside of the house. Get your heart going and get some of those beneficial brain molecules flowing through your system. Then, start on one of those tasks you've been avoiding.

How do I decide which task I should start first?

Does it really matter? Sometimes it does, a lot of times it doesn't. Most of the time, getting anything done is way better than getting nothing done. Just unload that dishwasher and think about how happy future-you will be when there's room for the dinner dishes later on. Even picking a low-stakes task will get you started in the right direction, because completing it will give you a little dopamine reward. That little reward will give you momentum to keep moving on to the next task.

If there is any task that has a time-bound sense of urgency attached to it, that might be a good one to start on. Or, is there an agenda item on your white board coming up that could use a little prepwork ahead of time? That's another place to start.

If you are really having trouble prioritizing you can . . .

Are you going to say "make a to-do list"?

Yeah. You can give it a shot. To-do lists actually can be very helpful in organizing what tasks you want to get done in the day. You don't have to let the things that need to get done swim around in your brain in the DMN space, pulling your attention away from getting any of the tasks done. If the list is held on a piece of paper or a planner or an app, it's not hogging memory resources in your brain. You can use that energy to actually do the things instead of trying to remember what things to do.

If to-do lists are so helpful, how come I can never finish one?

I suspect it's because your time-blindness issues lead you to unrealistically overload your to-do list. A common problem is that we get very optimistic about how much we can get done. We get so excited about making the list and remembering all the tasks we want to put on it that we forget to check the list against our task duration data (see above, in the time-blindness questions).

We have a tendency to make intricate, well-organized lists with annotations and subtasks. They are beautiful to look at and inspiring to behold. They are also physically impossible to complete in one day because we didn't bother to realistically assess how long each task will take. We also tend to neglect putting meals and rest on our lists. This can be a big mistake.

When you're making a to-do list, try to be realistic about how much of it you can actually get done. Also, give yourself permission to kick tasks down to tomorrow's list. And, maybe try making your list a little less pretty so you don't feel so bad if something doesn't get finished.

There are plenty of to-do list schemes, journaling techniques, and apps out there. I've heard of a bunch and forgotten them all, so I can't really recommend any particular system. My system is "write stuff down on a random scrap of paper and put that paper somewhere I'll see it often during the day."

How can I stay motivated to complete long-term projects?

I love long-term projects. I feel like I start long term-projects all the time. The beginning phase is so exciting! I can visualize how

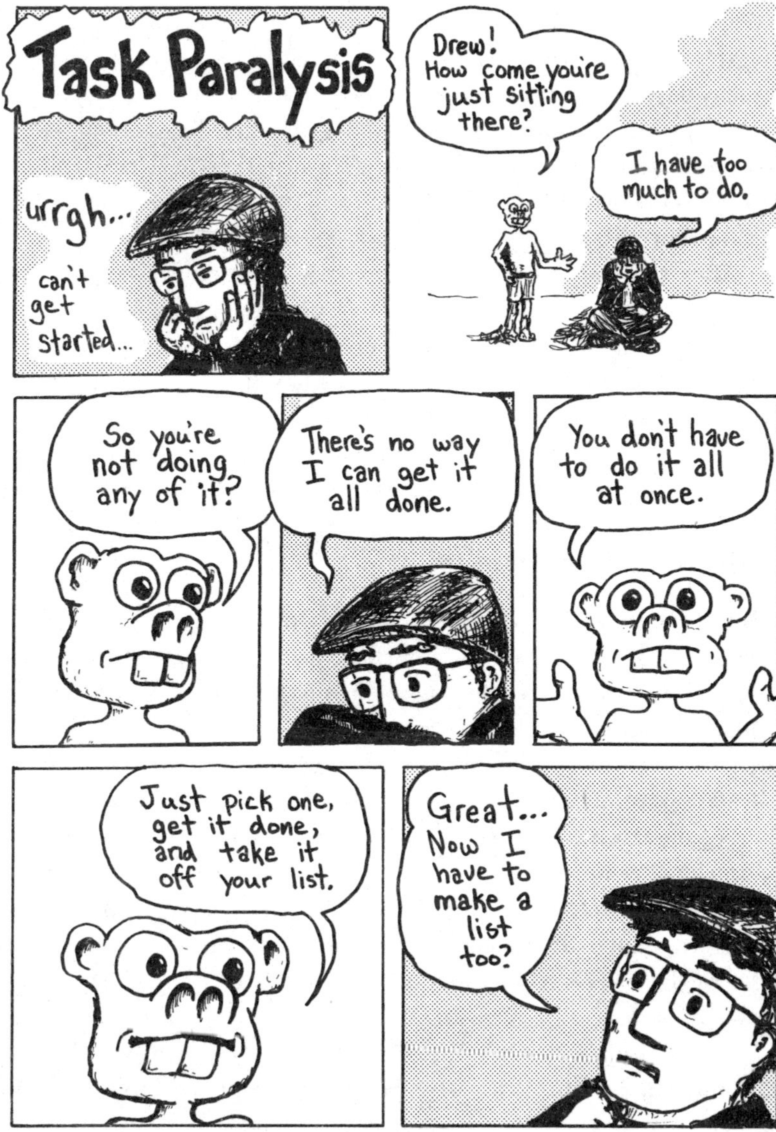
Task Paralysis
urrgh...
can't get started...
Drew! How come you're just sitting there?
I have too much to do.
So you're not doing any of it?
There's no way I can get it all done.
You don't have to do it all at once.
Just pick one, get it done, and take it off your list.
Great... Now I have to make a list too?

amazing the end product is going to be and how much it will enrich my life, or advance my career, or whatever. The first phase of any long-term project is usually a very DMN-dominated phase. We are actually daydreaming towards a purpose, and that's what our ADHD brains are really good at. A lot of times, this first phase includes price research and comparison shopping of materials, which can roll right into the one task the DMN and the TPN like teaming up for: buying stuff online!

After the buying of stuff, then comes the phase of actually having to do work on the project. This is where things tend to get bogged down in inaction and overwhelm. And a bit of guilt that we bought all this stuff that we probably have to return because there's no freaking way phase two's motivation is up to the task of meeting phase one's enthusiasm. But so many places charge a restocking fee that we better just get to it. Or keep the pile of supplies in the garage until it's time to move houses.

But it doesn't have to be this way.

What if it's a work thing my boss wants me to do?

That can present some of its own challenges, but also some perks. Like, hopefully, your employer is paying for all the necessary equipment and materials (unless you work in education . . . sorry teachers). And there is the external motivation from the boss that can add that motivating sense of urgency. It can be a mixed bag, but, largely, the motivation tips are the same for a self-directed project and an employer-directed project.

First, try not to be overwhelmed by the monumentality of taking on a huge job. Because every huge job can be broken down into manageable parts. I realized this when we were thinking about redoing our deck.

The house we live in came with an old, rotting wooden deck that, upon inspection, appeared to be held together by a mixture of dog hair and urine. We got an estimate for a redo from a contractor.

They wanted $18,000 for the job.

That was a lot more than we were able to pay. But we also knew that we really wanted to be able to enjoy our backyard without worrying someone's foot would go through the boards. We priced out the materials and came up with a figure of about $3,500. I worked for a school and had summers off. I had the time. I had the power tools. I was highly motivated by both the challenge and the thought of saving almost $15,000 dollars.

"I can redo the deck."

"Are you sure?" my wife asked. "It's a big job."

"Naw," I said. "It's just a lot of little jobs."

It was. A lot. Of little jobs. So many little jobs. I may have underestimated how many. Also, I underestimated how heavy those engineered deck boards can be. But I did it. One little dopamine burst at a time.

This technique is often called building a motivation bridge. The whole huge project can be represented as a plank bridge over a ravine. Each smaller task of the huge project is represented by the individual planks in the bridge. You don't have to be motivated to build the whole bridge, you only need to be motivated to place one plank at a time. As each plank in the project is put into place, you get a dopamine hit and a self-esteem boost. You can use the momentum from that boost to get started on the next plank. It builds and builds, and soon you've got the whole bridge done.

What if my project is not a physical thing like a bridge or a deck?

A lot of big jobs exist in an ephemeral world of work emails, video meetings, and cloud computing documents. It can be very hard to feel like you're making progress in the virtual world when your time-blindness, your quirky sense of object permanence, and your constantly refreshing working memory can no longer make sense of all the open browser tabs on your computer screen.

If this is the case, I suggest going analog. Have some sort

Side Quest: More about Motivation

I took an educational psychology course once upon a time, and one of the things that stuck with me was the idea of intrinsic versus extrinsic motivation. Intrinsic motivation is when the desire to do something comes from within yourself. Doing the thing satisfies an inner need that doesn't really have anything to do with anyone outside yourself. Extrinsic motivation is when you are doing the thing to fulfill a need or desire that exists outside of yourself. Your parents ask you to take out the trash. Your professor assigns a research paper. Your boss wants you to show up to work on time.

On those perfect days when we are at peace and in harmony with the world, intrinsic and extrinsic motivation are lined up with each other and working with synergistic add-on effects that boost our productivity in ways that artificially inflate everyone's expectations of what we can accomplish.

But, not every day is a perfect day.

On regular days in the real world, it is pretty common for there to be a bit of push and pull between intrinsic and extrinsic motivation. For a lot of people, it's a mild, grudging resistance that fades once the TPN gets going. For ADHDers, it can be a battle within themselves.

As has been mentioned before, the switches between activating the TPN and the DMN are very loose in the ADHD brain. The DMN is where intrinsic motivation has its summer home. If anything bumps an ADHDer from the TPN work on an externally assigned project and into the DMN, intrinsic motivation is going to go fishing for other projects to get excited about.

Meanwhile, on the extrinsic motivation front, things are getting desperate. The ADHDer's craving for connection can lead them toward an out-of-balance, people-pleasing urge. Fear of disappointing the project boss and feeling that rejection ratchets up the pressure. Add to it the anxiety of possibly disappointing a third party on an unrelated task because they overbooked their time (one part time-blindness, one part being thrown off by what they got done on that perfect day). It all teams up to throw their extrinsic motivation into an unfocused frenzy.

So, as you are using your tools, look for ways you can use them to bring extrinsic and intrinsic motivation into alignment.

of physical, real-world system of tracking your progress. While writing this book, I made a sticker chart. And I didn't just use any old Lisa Frank stickers, either. I used stickers that meant something to me. Most of my stickers came from artists at zine fairs and makers' markets. Some came in the mail with zines that were traded. They all spark with the joy of human connection as I put them on my chart. One sticker for every 1,000 words.

It doesn't have to be stickers. It could be LEGOs, or special rocks, or crudely gouged notches in the side of your desk. It could even be sitting in one of those browser windows, if that's your thing. The most important part is the meaning you give to celebrating each little accomplishment on the path to completing the huge project.

As of this point, I am so motivated to put stickers on the chart I can hardly wait to start writing my next book.

What about planners, calendars, and stuff?

Everyone loves to recommend daily planners, journals, calendars, apps, whatever. The problem is that daily planners can be the most boring things in the world. Calendars, same, unless it's a cool wall calendar with stuff you like on it. A boring organizational tool is not going to be used.

However, if you can trick out that planner into something you find entertaining, you might get some more value out of it.

My best, most useful calendars have always been the ones I drew myself. If I didn't make the calendar myself and hang it on the wall, odds are it's still on March 2020. But if I made it myself? Added illustrations and special icons for different important events? Implemented a weird color-coding scheme that only makes sense to me? You bet I used that calendar.

But that's me. I also have had a lot of luck using a passport sized notebook that fits in my shirt pocket. Sure, I draw a lot of weird gremlins in there and it's not necessarily in any particular page order, but sometimes just the act of writing something down is all I need to get it out of working memory and transferred to short-term memory. It has worked so very often. And, also, if all I remember is that I wrote it down, I've got the notebook in my pocket and I can look through it.

Some people like electronic organizational devices. And I get it. I've got some pretty sweet spreadsheets for certain things. I also have an accounting program that sends me reminders when it's time to check on zine consignments and things like that.

So, yeah. These tools can be great. But they have to be the tools that work for you. They have to be tools you are excited to use.

How do I make it so that everyday tasks aren't so painfully boring?

Boredom is definitely the enemy. I like to tell myself that I can't be bored if there's something to do. That doesn't always work. Actually, it usually makes me feel annoyed and tired. There are better ways:

- Gamify. Make games out of those tasks. Mary Poppins the hell out of all the boring things in life. Turn tidying up into an epic game of "the floor is lava." Anything on the carpet that's not a piece of furniture is going to be incinerated if you don't put it in its home in fifteen minutes. Make daily and weekly tasks worth points. See how many points you can add up in a day. If you want to get next-level, there are computer games and apps out there that bring the dynamics of a gaming experience to the regular, boring stuff.

- Try body doubling. The term *body doubling* is confusing because, when I first heard it, it made me think of mad scientist Frankenstein stuff. But in the ADHD sense, body doubling is really just having someone else around when you're having trouble staying on task. Having trouble getting off the couch? Call a friend to come over and work

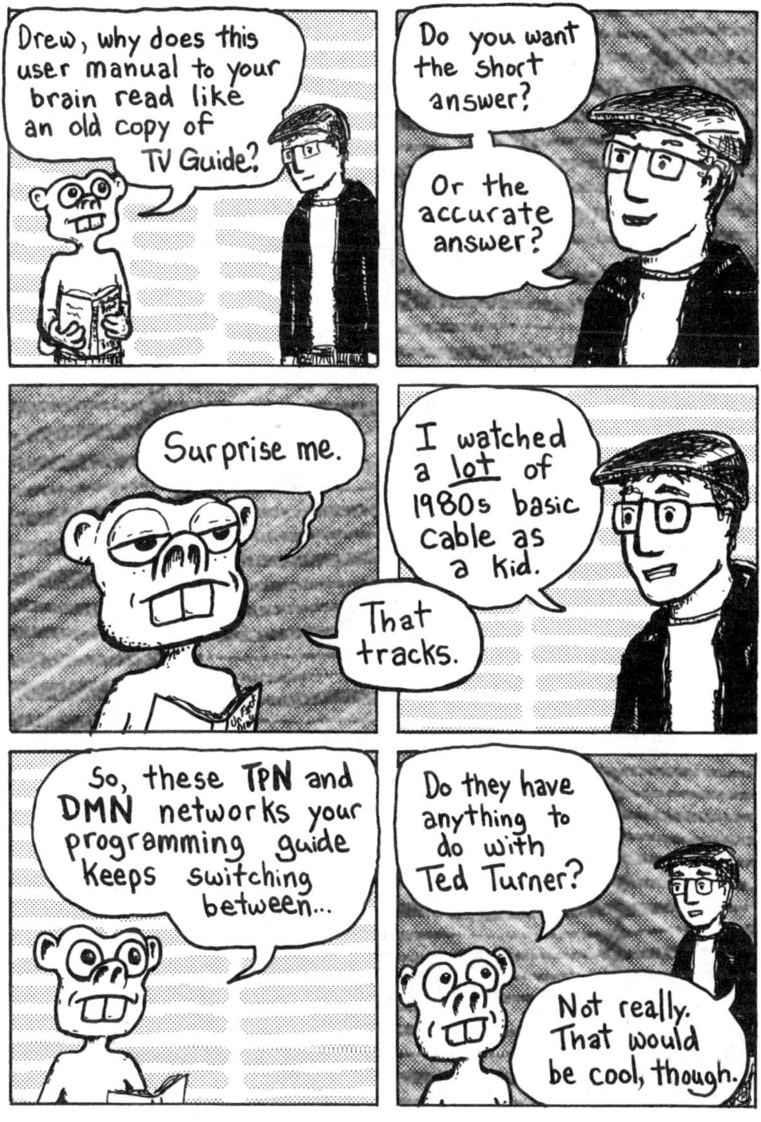
Drew, why does this user manual to your brain read like an old copy of TV Guide?
Do you want the short answer?
Or the accurate answer?
Surprise me.
I watched a lot of 1980s basic cable as a kid.
That tracks.
So, these TPN and DMN networks your programming guide keeps switching between...
Do they have anything to do with Ted Turner?
Not really. That would be cool, though.

on something while you do your thing. Or, if your friend is not into leaving the house, or they live in a different city, body doubling totally can be done over a voice or video call.

- Change the setting. Some tasks are more portable than others. With the portable ones, try taking them to a different room or outside. If you've got some tedious stuff to do on your laptop computer, try taking it to a park or a coffee shop.
- Get an accountability buddy. This is a scaled-up version of body doubling and is better for ongoing or long-term projects. Have someone you regularly check in with about your project. Have a scheduled chat with them at least once a month to talk about what you've gotten done and what you see the next steps being. This will inspire you to make some progress between check-ins. It's a good idea if it's a mutual arrangement where both participants are accountability buddies on each other's projects. Having an accountability buddy adds a measure of healthy extrinsic motivation to keep yourself going when your intrinsic motivation hits a lull.
- Schedule downtime. Make it part of your daily or weekly routine. If you have a busy week at work and you have a two-day weekend, go ahead and schedule yourself to be off duty for anything on Saturday. If your schedule doesn't fit the five on, two off pattern, schedule your downtime in a way that makes sense. But schedule it. Just have a time when your brain has absolute permission to not think about or do any of those boring everyday things. You need it. It'll pay off.

How can I avoid rejection crash (otherwise known as RSD)?

Okay. So, this is a big problem. Many ADHDers have some messed-up attachment histories where the people they counted on in their past for love, support, and guidance have repeatedly gotten on their ass for doing things wrong, for as long as they can remember. A lot of people on the internet have taken to heart the term *rejection sensitive dysphoria* as descriptive of the crippling emotional crash that can come out of the blue from something as simple as a comment about how their shirt is too wrinkled to wear to dinner.

But the jury is still out as to whether RSD is really its own thing.[9] Actually, if we're going to be accurate about our courtroom metaphor, the district attorney's office hasn't even put together their case yet. There hasn't been a trial or even an indictment. Rejection sensitive dysphoria isn't in the DSM-5. There hasn't been much real research into RSD, besides anecdotal evidence (which, admittedly, there is a lot of, if you follow ADHD TikTok at all).

There's something to RSD, but it isn't actually an officially diagnosable thing on its own.

My real reservation is that there are plenty of influencers who aren't as cautious as I am about using medical-sounding jargon to describe a problem while not actually offering any solutions. I'm kind of worried that people might lean on the RSD idea to justify dumping the blame onto someone or something outside their control when they're having a shitty time. I mean, yes, your shitty moment is real, and it's really shitty, but writing it off as someone triggering your RSD doesn't do a lot to help you move past it. And going down that path starts a behavioral pattern where no one around you is allowed to contradict you for fear of triggering your RSD. Not only is that super unhealthy for the other people in your life, it's too much like a *Twilight Zone* episode.

It's already been established that ADHDers have very strong emotions that can be difficult to regulate. That's why so many of us get misdiagnosed with mood disorders (especially women) before

9 Lindsay Weisner, PsyD, "Not Every Ailment We Experience Ends Up in the DSM," Psychology Today, September 25, 2024, https://www.psychologytoday.com/us/blog/the-venn-diagram-life/202409/is-rejection-sensitive-disorder-real-or-really-in-your-head.

getting a proper ADHD diagnosis. That's why so many of us have trouble with addiction, because we've tried to self-medicate our emotional volatility when the emotions were not actually the core problem.

Which is why I prefer the term *rejection crash.* Something happens. Someone says something or does something that drags up some old and deep emotions about how you feel about yourself and the world, and you just want to fall into a pit and disappear. Or worse. It's big. It's sudden. It's unpredictable. It's debilitating when it comes on. It's a total crash of your sense of self.

I don't know if you can avoid a rejection crash without doing some work on the feelings behind it. And that's where we really have to identify what this feeling is.

Now, my autistic part has a lot of trouble figuring out what I'm feeling. Alexithymia is a thing. It's taken me decades to really be able to decipher subtleties in my emotions beyond simple fear and excitement. One feeling-word I kept seeing in my research, especially as I was reading Richard Pink and Roxanne Emery's excellent book *Dirty Laundry,* was *shame.* So much of Roxanne's stories of her ADHD struggles revolved around shame. And my autistic side was like, "I'm not sure I feel shame. Maybe I need to learn more about what shame is."

Which, of course, led me to read Dr. Faith Harper's excellent book *Unfuck Your Shame.* Now, dear internet, please send all your @s to me as I tell you this. This shame thing is something I do feel. It's what I thought was RSD. But, no, for me, it's just a shame response. And I figured it out as I read Dr. Faith's book, where she is illuminating the difference between guilt and shame: "Guilt pushes us toward repair. By contrast, shame, because it activates disgust, tells us to remove ourselves from the situation in question. That we are the contaminant. That the repair in question *is our disappearance.*"

This is the rejection crash. It is the intense, ADHD-level shame that comes from feeling like such a failure that you just want to disappear.

So how do you avoid it? Um, well, about that . . .

So, if RSD is really a shame reaction, and I think it really is, we need to figure out what shame is (hint, read Faith's book). So, basically, shame is not a core emotion. It is not something that neurotypicals or ADHDers are born with. It's something we acquire later as we develop an understanding of self and how we fit into the social landscape we were born into. As such, shame looks different in different cultures. Some cultures have tools integrated into them for dealing with shame in a healthy way.

If you are reading this book in the original English, it is very likely that you were not born into one of those cultures. Western European cultures weaponized shame so hardcore during the Protestant Reformation and the Catholic Counter-Reformation that whole western economies run on the tension between guilt, shame, and the threat of eternal damnation. And that's not even taking into account the compounded effects of the later capitalist versus communist tensions of the Cold War Era . . . but I digress.

Basically, shame is an emotion that comes from looking at yourself and feeling that you fall short of the social expectations you had no choice in being born into.[10]

In summary, ADHDers, and the greater neurodivergent community in general, are often feeling like we're falling short of what the neurotypical-supremacist paradigm demands of us. This is the root of a lot of our shame because 80% of the people out there really struggle with understanding why we can't do things the way they expect us to. Their unthinking and instinctive go-to is to get frustrated and shout, harangue, bully, and demean us until we either

10 Not trying to step on any traditions that view karma and reincarnation as foundational components of human existence on earth. In fact, if you are well-versed in one of those traditions, you might have actually learned some better tools for processing and moving on from shame. Please shoot me some emails. Let's make a zine about it!

start approaching their standards, or we remove ourselves from their social landscape.

The urge to remove ourselves from society is a shame response. It is a reaction to how we've been told we fall short. It's a reaction to an unforgiving social landscape. Sadly, this urge for a neurodivergent person to remove themself from neurotypical society hits on a level beyond the garden variety awkwardness of letting a fart rip at church. Even more sadly, if you don't have buckets of money, there really aren't a lot of places to go. Content warning: this is a big part of why neurodivergents have a higher rate of unaliving themselves.

So, whether you call it a shame reaction, or a rejection crash, or RSD, the truth is, it can be a life-or-death problem. And western psychology has not done a lot of solid research on how to lessen shame in the individual. There's an old attitude, probably rooted in some Calvinist theological bullshit, that shame is a character defect rather than an emotional response based on shit that has happened to us that has wrecked our sense of self. Shame might get mislabeled as depression, and we might get some prescriptions for some fancy chemicals, but modifying the brain chemicals actually isn't very effective at helping us get over shame.

Which is probably why the TikTokers are screaming about needing their RSD taken seriously. The commonly prescribed pharmaceutical solutions are not working for them.

They didn't work for me, either, back in 1995. But I also didn't know what shame was. Or RSD. Or autism. Or ADHD. I just knew that I couldn't do the peopling the way other people did. The meds I did get prescribed, without much understanding of why I was having such intense feelings, just made me less inhibited and more of an asshole. In other words, I did more things that I was ashamed of.

Seeing as large swaths of western thought were letting me down, I had to get a little woo-woo.

I'll spare you my autodidact wizard travelog. It's not that interesting anyway. There's a few really simple core things you can do that don't require spending years in a monastery in Tibet or going to Findhorn like André Gregory (although I do highly recommend *My Dinner with André*, Louis Malle's 1981 film).

- First, accept who you are. Figure out who you are, how you work, what your quirks are, your strengths, and your weaknesses. All of it. Accept it. Accept that, at every point in your life, you are doing the best you can with what you have to work with. Those times in the past where other people made you feel like crap for the way you do things? You were actually doing the best you could.
- Second, dig a little deeper and figure out what you've been hiding from yourself. What are the urges, the fears, the doubts, and the past actions that your conscious mind does not want to own? What are the things in your shadow that you don't want to deal with?
- Third, have compassion for your shadow, the parts of yourself crammed into the darkest corner of your brain. Recognize them as part of your set of experiences. You wouldn't be who you are without that stuff. If you don't accept your shadow, how can you truly accept who you are? Sure. Some of that stuff may be scary as hell and you may need the help of a good therapist, coach, or spiritual guide to help you safely face it. Just try to make sure the person helping you out has a solid set of professional ethics and boundaries in place. Dealing with your shadow requires you to be vulnerable, so you don't want just any random amateur shaman coming in and rearranging your emotional furniture.
- Fourth, use the knowledge you've gained from your

shadow work. When a rejection crash comes on—and it will—recognize it, take a step back from whatever it is you're doing, get to a safe space, and allow yourself to feel it. While you're feeling it, remind yourself that feelings are transitory. If you allow yourself to feel a big, scary feeling, it will peak, and then it will diminish. As the intensity of the rejection crash ebbs, try to look for the real reason it came on. It usually has more to do with something that happened in your past rather than with the present.

- Most importantly, when the rejection crash comes, remember who you are, not who you think the world wants you to be. Shame works by diminishing your sense of self. Don't let it do that. If it helps, give the shame voice a name, like Ernie, and tell Ernie to back the fuck off when he starts up with his crap. What this is doing is reinforcing the fact that the shame is not actually a part of you. It's something that happens to you because of past negative social experiences. You don't have to let it take over.

Example time. Not very long ago, when we were getting ready to go somewhere, my wife expressed an opinion about the shirt I had picked out to wear. I am fairly fashion illiterate and I am often grateful for my wife's assistance. But every once in a while, it hits really hard. The rejection crash came on. I felt like I was losing my whole sense of individuality because I wanted to wear a shirt that could use some ironing.

It was a disproportionate response to what was happening. My wife was not trying to destroy my sense of self. In fact, she was actually trying to protect my sense of self by suggesting I try to look a little more put together when we left the house. But it hit me like a ton of manure. I had to lie down and put a pillow over my head for a few minutes.

I focused on breathing and reducing sensory input while I tried to figure out what was really going on inside me. For one, I was more tired than usual. We had a new baby in our lives and that had upended all the routines. That right there made me a little more raw and vulnerable than usual. On top of that, I was feeling the echoes of several moments of wardrobe criticism from my past. Beginning with the itchy clothes I was supposed to wear to church as a kid, to whatever the fuck was going on with running shorts in the 1970s. To the girl in seventh grade who stopped me in the hallway and had a lot to say about how I wore the same windbreaker zipped up all the way every day, even into the 90-degree springtime temperatures in Tucson, Arizona. To the time a coworker pointed out my eccentric choice to wear a plaid shirt with striped shorts. All of these were moments of wardrobe-related shame from the distant past, but they all came riding in on that ton of manure the rejection crash had dumped on me.

Being able to identify where all these feelings came from let me recognize that none of the feelings came from what my wife had said about my shirt being wrinkly. I was able to feel the feelings and let them pass. I was also able to come out of turtle mode, change my shirt, and go on to enjoy an evening with someone who loves me very much.

Like I said, this is a really tame example. I have much worse ones that have happened with my mom that I'm only just starting to figure out. (Sorry, mom.) But I will say this. Since I started stimulant ADHD meds, it's been so much easier to get through some triggering situations without having the full-blown rejection crash. Maybe this means there is something to the idea of RSD as a component of ADHD. Or maybe it just means that the stimulant meds for ADHD are helpful in many arenas of ADHD life beyond just focus.

How do I deal with feeling burned out?

We feel burned out when we've used up all our energy reserves. This is very easy for ADHDers to do, because we often get so wrapped

Side Quest:

Rejection and Recognition

As much shade as I throw at the term *rejection sensitive dysphoria*, it was actually coined by a medical professional, Dr. William Dodson, who has written about it in the pages of *ADDitude* on many occasions. Again, I'm not discounting the experience, just discounting the way social media influencers like to use RSD as a free pass not to deal with their shame issues.

In counterpoint, Dr. Edward Hallowell and Dr. John Ratey, also frequent fliers in the pages of *ADDitude*, like to emphasize that ADHD traits very often come in pairs with a positive for every negative. For example, the ADHDer's difficulty in remaining focused on the main thing in front of them also means they are able to see important details in the periphery that most people don't notice. Dr. Hallowell and Dr. Ratey like to help their patients, and their readers, find ways to leverage the positives in ways that mitigate the negatives. In the case of rejection sensitive dysphoria, they suggest in a 2019 webinar available on *ADDitude*'s website[1] that there is an equally powerful counter to RSD they call "recognition responsive euphoria." Basically, by getting into a habit of recognizing your successes, and being around people who recognize your successes, you can feel like a damn rockstar and perform a whole lot better in many aspects of your life where you otherwise struggle.

It might sound a little hokey, but there's something to it. Coming from working in educational settings with kids who have all kinds of struggles, it's widely accepted that best practice is giving kids six positives for every negative piece of feedback. It's really hard to pull off. Especially since some of these kids can be *super* assholes. But, in my experience, providing those positives works.

1 Edward Hallowell, MD, " 'The Flip Side of Rejection Sensitive Dysphoria: How to Tap Into ADHD Energy and Motivation' [Video Replay & Podcast 278]," February 14, 2025, https://www.additudemag.com/webinar/recognition-responsive-euphoria-adhd-podcast-278/.

up in something that we'll forget to eat or take breaks. We also often find ourselves burning the midnight oil because of our tendency to procrastinate on tasks until we feel a sense of urgency about them.

Ideally, employing the strategies discussed in the last two sections can help prevent burnout. Realistically, though, it takes time to get all those strategies in place. You can't implement them all at once. If you try to do too much too fast, you risk causing burnout. It's another one of those ADHD double-edged gift/curse conundrums.

So, be kind to yourself. Accept that not everything can fall into place all at the same time. Notice when you are overextending yourself. Try to be aware of those moments when you suddenly feel compelled to take on another project. Do you really have the energy for it? Or are there other things you are trying to avoid by taking on something new? Try to monitor and budget your energy realistically (again, hard to do and requires implementing other strategies, so take it easy).

Don't chase yourself in circles trying to avoid burnout. Instead, build downtime into your life. If you have no idea how much downtime you need, start with taking one day a week.

Set aside one day a week as a day where you don't have to do anything on any to-do lists. Let your partner, family, or housemates know this is a strategy you are actively employing. Ask them to help you out by letting you opt out of anything that might come up on your down day. You're not being lazy or inconsiderate. You're recharging your batteries so you'll have more to work with on the other days.

If you find yourself antsy and ready to do something after a couple hours of sanctioned rest on a downtime day, excellent! Your batteries have recharged. Go ahead and take care of some tasks. Or go to the movies with your favorite human. Use what you learned about how long it took to recharge for future scheduled downtimes.

Of course there will be a lot of varying factors. Not every week is the same, and it is sometimes very difficult to carve out downtime. But if you are at the point of burnout, you need it. Hopefully, by becoming mindful of your energy levels and your threshold of overwhelm, you can be able to preemptively build in appropriate downtime before the burnout point. By doing this, you should be able to decrease the amount of downtime you need to schedule. Recharging before you're fully burned out is much more efficient than recovering from a critical battery failure.

FOR PARENTS OF ADHD STUDENTS

In this section, I'm going to walk you through some of the tough things you're probably already living with. How to navigate school as a parent of an ADHDer. What you can honestly expect from the school system. And how to get okay with the fact that the emphasis on academic success really needs to take a backseat. It's much more important that your ADHD kids feel good about themselves as human beings, rather than overfocusing on what their math scores are.

What do parents need to know about school?

School is a fact of life in our world. The dominant paradigm says that kids need to go to school. There's also a heavy emphasis on going on to advanced studies after high school. There is a bizarre, yet ubiquitous, undertone in American culture that says if a kid can't make it in college, they might as well go die in a hole. And that message starts getting drilled into kids when they're in kindergarten.

There is something to be said for having goals and values and high expectations. Yes. We want our kids to dream big. Unfortunately, the way the system is set up, there's really only one variety of dream that gets openly validated: the variety of dream that requires a college degree to attain.

Now, I'm not saying this to discourage parents from sending their kids to school. I actually value education very much and have spent fifteen years of my life working in schools. I believe that schools are an important, foundational part of our society. Public schools are the smallest units of governmental civic engagement, and as such, have the most direct impact on everyday, real people.

We can't get rid of school. But what we can do is get more real about what the mission of schools is.

The number one mission of schools is not to send kids to college: it's to give them the skills to participate in the adult world. In the early twentieth century when the progressive movement was creating the modern school system, a big part of the mission of schools was to make sure the children of immigrants knew enough English to understand their bosses in the factories when they went to work after eighth grade. Not everyone was expected to go to high school, let alone college.

This system—designed to help create an industrially homogenized workforce—is way overdue for an update. Unfortunately, the system is still tied to the metrics of industrial output. Try as we might, we just can't get away from the idea that schools need standards and every single human child should be able to meet those standards. It's a noble ideal. But the system really only works well for one type of brain.

Neurodivergent children of all strands find struggles in school. The most important thing a parent of a child with ADHD can do is recognize the depth of those struggles and remove some of the pressure to conform to unrealistic standards.

Do I need to get special education services for my ADHD child?

Maybe. While access to a "free and appropriate public education" (FAPE) is enshrined into federal law in the United States, the slippery word in that terminology is *appropriate.* Appropriate to whom and for what?

Across the United States, the answer to this question can vary quite a bit. I've worked in schools in two states, Arizona and Oregon. I've had experiences in several different kinds of public education environments, from district schools to charter schools to after-school programs run by agencies outside of the traditional school system. The results vary in how the law is applied and what each agency's collective approach is.

It blew my mind when I came to Portland Public Schools from the Tucson Unified School District. At my interview to be a paraeducator, I described the high school program I had previously worked in and that I would like to find something similar. The administrator interviewing me basically said, "We don't have that here."

That being said, in spite of administrative directives and overwhelming bureaucratic bullshit, there are superheroic special education teachers in every dysfunctional educational system. People are drawn to working in special education out of a passion for doing something meaningful and helpful in the world. A lot of special education staff are neurodivergent themselves (whether they know it or not) and come with tremendous empathy for the kids who have the same kinds of struggles they did.

At the same time, it is a high-burnout profession. Some of the most promising special educators get burned out early on and either switch careers or resign themselves to a life of doing what they can to stay on top of the paperwork. Even worse, there are times when the most dedicated crusaders for their students get actively chased out of the profession by administrators who are tired of being constantly challenged by them.

This doesn't mean that special education is an overall horrible situation. It just means buckle up and be ready to do what you can to help your kid through the limitations of the system. Appreciate the limitations of the people who work with your kid in the system. Do your best to build positive and open communication with the teachers and the administrators who work with your kid. If they can't reciprocate the positive and open communication with you, it might be time to bring in a consultant.

Side Quest:

Paperwork

Just to point out the obvious. A special education teacher who is also an ADHDer is very likely to have empathy, intuition, and a personal mission of helping neurodivergent kids become successful adults. However, ADHD educators are also very likely to become overwhelmed with the job, drown in paperwork, lose track of important meetings, fall behind on data collection, and suffer from imposter syndrome and frequent rejection crashes. As much as school districts go through the motions of following special education law, when it comes to an employee asking for accommodations under ADA (the Americans with Disabilities Act), the school district HR teams are really good at finding the legal loopholes that let them say no.

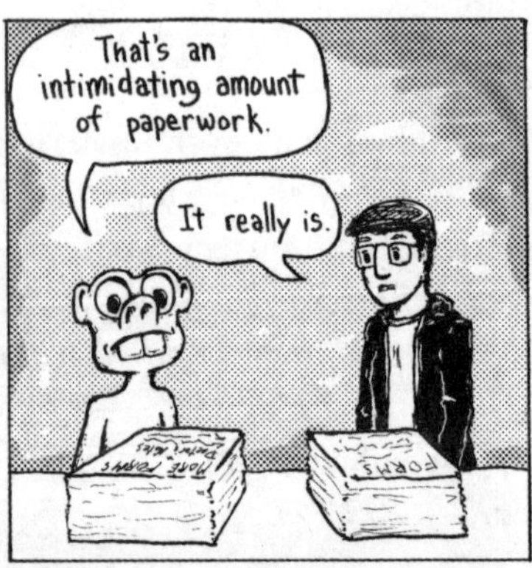

I've worked with some students whose ADHD symptoms were so profound they were put on an IEP (Individual Education Plan) before they entered kindergarten. Other students get identified later as a pattern of academic and behavioral problems appear. And some students don't get identified, often the inattentive-type ADHDers, because they don't have the behavioral problems that often fast-track the intervention process.

And none of that information really speaks to what these individual kids actually needed.

What all kids really need is involved adults who care about them. Getting on an IEP does increase the amount of adults the student works with in school. Maybe that increase is only by one, the special education teacher. Maybe the school is fortunate

continued...

enough to have classified paraprofessionals and educational assistants that can increase that number a bit. (Unfortunately, the classified staff are the lowest-hanging fruit when budget cuts come around. And they always come around.) An IEP can also direct some ADHD-specific accommodations like specialized lessons in study skills and organization, extra time to complete assignments, preferential seating, access to an alternative location for testing, sensory items (fidgets) to help burn off extra energy, and, if you're lucky, an adult that can work with them one-to-one or in a small group during times of the school day they have more trouble focusing.

So the real question is, what does your child really need to be successful in school? Is an IEP needed for the school to be able to provide these accommodations, or will a Section 504 plan suffice?

What is the difference between an IEP and a 504?

An IEP is a document that is required under the Individuals with Disabilities in Education Act (IDEA). This is the federal law in the United States that governs how special education works in American public schools. When a student is determined to have a disability that qualifies for special education services, they get an IEP written according to the guidelines in IDEA. IDEA is pretty strict in how eligibility is determined. Not only does there have to be a disability, it has to be shown that the disability has a negative effect on the student's educational success.

Not only does the IEP spell out the accommodations and modifications the student will receive, it also includes goals for the student and the required progress monitoring to keep track of how well the student is doing meeting those goals. An IEP is an imposing document that is often written in a stilted and highly technical way to satisfy any legal challenges that may come up in court.

ADHD itself does not have its own IEP disability category the way autism, deafness, and blindness do. It falls under the other health impaired (OHI) category. It's hard to prove that ADHD in itself is causing the student's educational difficulties. Most ADHDers who have IEPs also have another disability, often a learning disability or speech impairment, that qualifies them for special education eligibility.

However, many students with an ADHD diagnosis have no problem qualifying for a 504 plan.

The 504 plan is named after Section 504 of the Rehabilitation Act of 1973. This section of federal law has a lower barrier for establishing that a disability is limiting a child's ability to learn in an educational setting. 504 accommodations include anything that doesn't require a special education teacher to administer or direct it. In general, if a student only requires a couple minor accommodations to be able to learn in the regular classroom, a 504 is the plan for them.

A 504 plan is not as robust as an IEP. It lists accommodations to be provided and who is providing them, but it does not include goals, progress monitoring, or a transition plan for after high school. Also, a 504 plan does not necessarily provide access to special education paraprofessionals. If said parapro happens to be scheduled to push-in to the same general education classroom to provide accommodations for a student on an IEP that are similar to another student's 504 plan, they might be able to work with both in a small group. More likely, it will be up to the gen-ed teacher to scramble to get it done.

Fun fact: Section 504 applies only to public schools. IDEA applies to students in private schools as well as public schools. Does this mean those fancy private schools have their own special education staff? I wouldn't bet on it. The special education staff at the nearest public school are often required to serve the private school students. Is this the best possible arrangement? What do you think?

That being said, there are some private schools that are founded expressly to serve certain populations of disabled students. Because these schools can focus on their core mission without all the other requirements put upon public schools, they can have some wonderful results. America is a land of golden opportunities so long as you have enough gold to pay for them.

Of course, as with everything else in the American education system, your results may vary.

Side Quest:

The Thirteen Disability Categories Covered by IDEA

- Autism Spectrum Disorder
- Blindness
- Deafness
- Emotional Disturbance
- Hearing Impairment
- Intellectual Disability
- Multiple Disabilities
- Orthopedic Impairment
- Other Health Impaired
- Specific Learning Disability
- Speech or Language Impairment
- Traumatic Brain Injury
- Visual Impairment

How helpful are these plans, really?

The plans can be really helpful if they are written well, implemented well, and amended as needed in response to the realities of what's going on. Of all the frustrations that come with working in special education, one of the unmitigated joys is watching individual students progress and grow over the years.

Is it because of the IEP or in spite of it? It's hard to say. I have worked mostly as a paraeducator, with very little say in the development of IEPs. And, these days, IEPs are often digital documents on a software platform that many classified (i.e., non-licensed) staff, like paraeducators, don't have access to.

In my practice, I have found it much more helpful to get to know who the student is, become their partner in problem-solving, and help them learn how to deal with the challenges of the school environment. I do follow the direction of the special education teacher on how to implement accommodations and deliver instruction, but I'm always looking for a way to help with the more intangible aspects of navigating the complex and confusing world of school.

What is the most important school-based intervention?

The single most important intervention for any student is connection.

Whether it's intentional or not, ADHDers get a lot of negative reinforcement about what kind of student they are. Before being identified as ADHD, and even afterwards, they get a lot of feedback from others at school about how they are doing things wrong. This feedback comes from school staff and fellow students. Sometimes it comes from the parents of fellow students.

There is some special magic about being a child with ADHD that makes them lightning rods for negative attention. Especially for those with the hyperactive/impulsive flavor. The blurts, the sudden movements, the big energy—all these have the effect of causing the teacher (and other students) to give them behavior reminders far more often than neurotypical students. And ADHDers are very aware of the fact that they get these reminders more often. And those reminders are painful to receive, especially at those times when they are rooted in how excited and motivated a student is to participate.

ADHD students feel isolated, incompetent, and misunderstood. They can feel like they are forced to participate in a system that was never designed for them. This feeling is absolutely valid. The American school system was specifically designed for the education of neurotypical white children. The very idea that public schools should be a place for all children to be able to access equally really didn't become a thing until the Civil Rights Movement. And for someone with an invisible disability like ADHD, that's an idea that only exists on paper.

You can quote 1970s-era special education law to a ten-year-old all day long, but that's not going to make them feel like school is actually a place for them.

What they need is this: to know that there are adults at the school who are truly on their side. They need their strengths recognized and their contributions valued.

I have been fortunate enough to spend most of my education career at a school where most of the staff work really hard to do this. It is not easy. And when there is a teacher that isn't good at it, it really shows. Kids get a very real opinion about which teachers and staff members hate them. The adults in question might not actually hate the student, but it's what the student feels. And if the adult doesn't recognize the strength of that child's feelings and isn't able to do the work necessary to change that perception, they might as well write that student off.

That's not to say the adults at school need to roll over and give ADHD students carte blanche to indulge every impulse. My friend Greta West, who is a school speech and language pathologist, as well as a staunch advocate for her own neurodivergent children, says one of the most important things to do as an educator and a parent is to "teach [the student] how to be accountable but still have their back." No one is arguing that kids don't need to learn how to be accountable for their actions. We just have to remember that they are still kids and, as kids, they need adults who can be partners with them in solving problems that are way too huge for them to solve on their own.

How do we make sure connection happens at school?

This is a toughie. IEP teams like to write IEPs with measurable goals towards which they can monitor the progress. But how can anyone measure such an internal and subjective thing as connection? I'm sure behavioral scientists can give us a list of tools for measuring such things across large demographic groups. But on the individual, granular level of one student? Giving a kid a research-backed screening questionnaire on how connected they feel to their social surroundings is probably not going to give reliable results. In fact, using such a measuring tool might actually backfire and cause the student to feel even more singled-out and isolated than they did at baseline.

Of course, no one on the IEP team is going to argue that connection and integration with the social environment of school is not worthwhile. They're just going to have trouble writing this into a progress goal in a way that doesn't feel insulting and absurd.

It can be done. And it must be done, because that sense of connection with the humans around students is what provides meaning to all the other educational goals we have for them.

One way to do this is to have a staff member be a check-in/check-out person for the student. The check-in/check-out happens at the beginning of the day and at the end of the day. It can be a very formal thing where there's a worksheet that describes a specific (easily and unequivocally measurable) academic or behavioral goal. The staff member and student discuss strategies for meeting that specific goal, while also checking in on more nebulous things like how they're feeling, whether they liked breakfast, how things were on the bus, how they slept, etc. Little points of relatable, human connection that send the message that the staff member cares about how the student is doing as a person.

It is important that this check-in/check-out person is consistent. This is really about relationship building. If the staff member who does the check-in/check-out has a role where they often get called off to deal with emergent issues at the check-in/check-out time, this will undermine the goal of building connection.

Another way of building connection in the school is by asking the school to hold a neurodivergent student affinity group. Many schools already have affinity groups for minority students and for LGBTQIA+ students and allies. Sometimes there is even an additional funding stipend for the adults who facilitate the groups. One of the most rewarding things I got to do this past year was to lead a neurodivergent group at the school I worked at. The kids really appreciated having a space to meet once a week and let down all their guards and be real about the quirky things their brains do sometimes.

My school also had some parent advocates who started a monthly after-school meet-up for families of neurodivergent students.

Groups?! Doesn't my invisibly disabled child have a right to privacy concerning their invisible disability?

Yes. Of course. As a matter of human decency and as a matter of the Family Educational Rights and Privacy Act. FERPA is the law that, similar to HIPAA in the medical professions, binds school employees from irresponsibly broadcasting personal information about the students they work with. If you do not want your child's special education services and eligibility discussed with anyone outside the IEP team and school administration, you have that right to privacy.

Even beyond special education matters, there are so many

reasons why family privacy needs to be respected. People are judgy as hell and kids need to be protected from that bullshit. Bullying happens. Discrimination happens. Stressful parental custody issues that aren't anybody else's business happen. I understand and respect the parents' rights to keep a tight and heavy lid on whatever information they need to.

However, I am also a huge believer in people feeling good about who they are. It's really hard for a kid to develop a positive self-image and feel genuine connection with others when they feel they have to hide a part of themselves. So often, ADHDers exhaust themselves trying to pretend to be normal that they don't have any reserves left when the mask inevitably slips. This failure to appear normal—the failure to keep their secrets hidden behind the FERPA wall—makes them feel like they are failures at being human.

If families feel comfortable being open about ADHD, it can be liberating. It removes a source of shame and gives it the opportunity to become a source of pride. When ADHD students are able to talk about neurodivergence openly, they end up finding neurodivergent friends. They end up gaining neurotypical allies. They get more sources of connection that help them be more grounded and involved in the world around them.

Is it realistic to expect my child's school to be able to provide that point person for connection?

Sadly, no. But you really should push for it anyway. Cite the ACES study, quote Mr. Rogers, refer them back to the mission statement of their school district. All of those will reinforce the core idea that all children need positive adult connections to thrive. School budgetary constraints and ridiculously inflated teacher workloads are the main obstacles. The system is at odds with the reality of human needs. None of the humans involved want to deprive a child of human connection. They just have too much on their plates to keep up with it all.

Being a demanding pain in the ass at the IEP meeting makes sure everyone else on the team keeps your kid on their radar.

But you might be lucky. There is a chance that your school actually does have enough support staff to facilitate a meaningful check-in/check-out system or run an affinity group.

Why don't schools have enough support staff?

It really depends on the school district, their funding sources, their strategy of community engagement, and their overall staffing levels.

One of the biggest bargaining points during teacher contract negotiations is reducing class sizes and increasing support staff. Unfortunately, the result is often a compromise where the district offers stipends to teachers whose classes are over capacity . . . and classified support staff get cut in order to pay for it.

Some schools have super active PTSOs (Parent-Teacher-Student Organizations, or PTAs, if you're old school) that are able to fundraise to pay for a staff position or two. This really depends on the neighborhood and the fundraising rules of the school district in question.

Special education staffing gets a little different. There is federal money tied to implementing IDEA (but not Section 504). Depending on the level of disability and the special education programs at a school, that federal money could pay for some special education paraprofessionals. However, it is very difficult to get a paraprofessional allocated for one student with ADHD. Paraprofessionals are more often assigned to programs that serve students with more visible disabilities or orthopedic accessibility needs. There's also a lot of variation to this. Some school districts have moved to full inclusion models, with more parasupport in every classroom.

Why does my kid keep getting suspended?

Kids with ADHD, especially the hyperactive-impulsive flavor, seem to be lightning rods for conflict. If there is trouble happening anywhere near a school setting, the ADHD child will be involved in it.

My dad, who doesn't have an ADHD diagnosis—but he's my dad, so odds are . . . Anyway, he has a lot of stories about getting into trouble with the nuns in Catholic school back in the 1950s. One he likes to tell is about how he was sent to go wash his mouth out with soap so often, they stopped sending a nun with him to make sure he did it. They didn't need to. He had the routine down. He was a rule follower. But he also was impulsive and had picked up a lot of cussing from his older brothers. When he got into a disagreement with someone, the blue streak would come streaming out.

It's very similar to the pattern I've seen with some students with ADHD. They are doing their best in class. They care about the rules. They are trucking along just fine. And then the kid in the seat behind them whispers a rude comment or joke. The ADHD student is not able to stifle their laughter, nor are they able to contain their retort, which comes out at a playground-level voice. The whole class gets set off in a gigglefest that takes the teacher a couple minutes to defuse.

And who gets called out on inappropriate behavior? Not the student who whispered the original comment. The ADHD student catches the flack. And when they try to point out why they did, they are further chastened for not being able to control themselves and talking back to the teacher.

It's a condition of their disability that they are not always able to control themselves. And they are being publicly shamed for it. Whereas the whispering student was able to control themselves, quietly engage in inappropriate behavior, and melt back into the rest of the tittering classroom without an individual reprimand.

Every time this happens with the ADHD student, it's another wound to their self-esteem. It's another piece of damning evidence that, no matter how hard they try to be good, they just get in trouble anyway. It makes them question whether it's even worth it to try anymore. And it takes away some of their resilience for the next time a conflict comes up. And because they're a kid, and they're already stretched pretty close to the breaking point, the next conflict might end up with punches thrown instead of just words.

This pattern repeats over and over. The blurts and comments in class get phone calls home. The fights result in suspensions. The suspensions result in trouble at home. The hole keeps getting dug deeper and deeper.

This student needs that human connection lifeline desperately. Someone that can listen to them, hear them, believe them, and believe in them.

What about social skills education and bullying?

All kids need help learning social skills, but for some reason, schools only assign social skills lessons to neurodivergent students. Some lip service was given to increasing Social Emotional Learning (SEL) when kids came back to school after the COVID shutdowns. But then, after a couple months, the school administrators got back to harping on the Common Core Standards. There's only so much time. Some teachers are very good at integrating SEL instruction with everything else they have to do. Some aren't. This is life.

Bullying is a problem in this world, no doubt. I have been blessed with the right combination of autistic traits that make me pretty oblivious to when bullying behavior has been directed at me. I tend to just get confused and withdraw in a way that doesn't give the bully the reaction they're looking for. Most of the time they move on and bother someone else. I am also sufficiently old that it's really not an issue anymore.

For kids growing and learning in the constantly shifting social dynamics of an arbitrarily assembled group of their same-aged peers, it's bound to be a mess.

A lot of times, ADHD students feel like they are being bullied. Sometimes ADHD students get identified as being bullies. It is

Side Quest:

Connection

In my old job as a special education paraeducator, I made it my mission to connect with as many students as possible, not just the ones on the special education caseload.

Part of it is just good professional practice. Interacting with all the students in a classroom makes it less stigmatizing when I am helping a student that's on the caseload. I'm seen by the students as an adult who helps out everyone, rather than an adult who helps out the special needs kids. This is also a good way to address family privacy concerns by making it less obvious which students are getting special education services.

Another part is, I developed pretty good intuition about which students would end up on the caseload. If I could develop a positive relationship with them early on, it helped us both in the long run. They may not end up qualifying for services, but our neurodivergence recognition software clicks, and they know I can be a safe, understanding adult who can help with social weirdsies on the playground.

Speaking of the playground, paraprofessionals often get tapped for recess and cafeteria supervision duty. It's good to get to know as many of the kids as possible.

In addition, as a self-advocate, I do not hide my neurodivergencies from the kids. I talk about being neurodivergent. I talk about how my brain gets stuck sometimes, or gets extra unstuck other times. I'm open about moments where something has overwhelmed me and caused my "cranky voice" to come out. I provide myself as a role model and an example of how a neurodivergent person can be an adult. It has been one of the biggest successes of my career that so many students have seen me as someone who can understand them when it feels like no one else can. All because I'm not afraid of being real, vulnerable, and genuine with them.

This is connection.

almost always confusing to them as to what the distinction is.

The standard package of social skills is very compliance-based. The lessons usually describe a set of rules prescribed for certain social situations. But then the kids with the special ed social skills class see the other kids breaking those rules all the time. Social skills, it turns out, are very dynamic and situational. Not everyone follows the script. In fact, people who don't follow the script can get better results in certain situations.

A lot of kids with ADHD see this disconnect and conclude that the rules don't apply all the time. But when should the rules apply? What are the situations? And so begins an entire socratic dialog about what-is-justice-anyway.

This isn't to say social skills education is a waste of time. Just that it is often delivered in an unrealistic and ableist way that leads some kids to reject it outright.

What skills should I ask the IEP team to focus on?

There are some definite skill areas where ADHDers can benefit from extra practice and scaffolding:

- time management
- organization of materials
- regulation of body energy

Every student is going to have struggles with all of these to some degree, so it should be possible to implement some simple interventions without making it a spectacle.

Time Management

Time management can be supported in lots of ways:

- Modeling. The teacher most likely already has a daily schedule posted in the classroom. Making it a normal part of classroom discussion to refer to the schedule provides a simple reinforcement of the passage of time. ADHDers can easily slip into the DMN mode of timeless contemplation. Referring to the schedule is throwing them a line to help pull them back into TPN.

- Task duration estimation. Either in the whole class or in small groups, a teacher can lead the students to discuss how much time they think certain tasks take to complete. This shouldn't be a one-off lesson, but a continual practice that helps students create an awareness of what can be accomplished in a certain block of time. One issue ADHDers come up against is getting frozen in unproductivity if they know there is something important coming up later in the day. They become so focused on being ready for the later event that it is very difficult to initiate other tasks before then. Time estimation practice for long tasks can help them know whether it's realistic to start and finish a task within the time available.
- Checklists. Simple checklists that delineate the steps of an assignment. Oftentimes, an ADHDer will get lost thinking about the whole of the project before they even begin. They'll get stalled-out thinking about the end stages before they even put their name at the top of the paper. A checklist helps give a physical structure to anchor the student to the steps of the process.
- Timers. Timers can be helpful. Or they can be one more distracting thing. A timer that informs the whole class about the duration of an activity may be more helpful than an individual task time on the student's desk. If a student is able to handle their own timer, the pomodoro method of alternating a set amount of work with a set amount of brain break time can be very helpful.

Organization of Materials

The organization of materials is the constant bugbear of the student's backpack and desk. Unfortunately, the most commonly used strategy in schools is a big, fat three-ring binder with multiple sections. Any organizational scheme that requires more than three steps to utilize is going to be troublesome for an ADHDer. In the case of the binder, there's opening the binder, turning to the right section, finding the right sheet of paper you need, opening the rings, taking the sheet out (or putting it in), and closing the rings again. That's six steps that need to be managed in the student's working memory. And that's on top of whatever it is they're supposed to do with that sheet of paper. While a neurotypical child might be able to chunk the whole binder routine into one or two steps, the ADHDer is much more likely to miss a part along the way. Missing any one of those six steps of managing the binder sets the student up for disaster later.

A simpler system of individual folders for each subject will be much easier for an ADHDer to handle. Even better if they are different colors.

Having other materials stored in open bins that are easy to visually scan can be very helpful. It's easy to see right off the bat what's in the right place and what's in the wrong place.

Having an enclosed or obscured compartment under the desktop is liable to become a hoarder's nest of crumpled papers, overdue library books, broken pencils, and sometimes food.

Regular desk and backpack clean-out times can also be necessary.

Regulating Body Energy

Regulating body energy is basically giving the student opportunities to burn off the restlessness before it becomes a problem in class. Believe it or not, it can be uncomfortable, to the point of being physically painful, for some neurodivergent students to sit still for long periods of time. Hopefully your IEP team includes an occupational therapist. OTs have great strategies for helping kids integrate their minds and bodies into the classroom environment.

- A daily sensory routine can do wonders. It doesn't take long. All it needs is a space and a staff member to facilitate. Sensory routines vary depending on the student and what equipment is available. Exercises that involve balance engage the cerebellum in a way that benefits ADHDers' ability to self-regulate and helps with executive function. Exercises that cross the midline (right hand touches left knee, for example, or twisting arms into a pretzel position) helps coordinate signals between both hemispheres of the brain. Exercising the brain helps it drive the body.
- Sensory cushions on stretchy bands for classroom chairs can give students some relief and an opportunity to quietly wiggle while still being engaged in class.
- Fidgets. Fidgets are very popular. Some of them are a little bit too fun. It can be tricky to find the right object that can be a helpful tool without becoming an unhelpful distraction. And this will vary from day to day, student to student. The important thing is to find what works.

There are also some whole-class strategies you can suggest the teacher put into place. These may be outside of your control as a parent, but you can totally bring them up at IEP meetings:

- Take whole-class movement breaks.
- Chunk seatwork into twenty-minute segments with physical transitions between segments (getting materials, water breaks, turn and tells).
- Get class to recess on time! (Too often, I've seen teachers hold classes inside until everyone can be quiet and in line. And guess who gets the blame from the rest of the class

for holding up the show? The students with ADHD who are at the living ends of their ropes from sitting still.)

Does the IEP include traditional mental health therapy?

Not really. The IEP's function is to help a student successfully access academic instruction in the school setting. While there sometimes are wraparound mental health services offered by an outside provider at school sites, these are generally not within the purview of the IEP. (There are always exceptions, especially for students whose primary educational disability is identified as "Emotional Disturbance." Someone else is going to have to write that book.)

Ideally, this kind of school-based therapist will be in good communication with the IEP team, and even invited to IEP meetings. This does require parental consent and release of information (ROI) documents to ensure FERPA and HIPAA rights are protected.

Similarly, therapy received outside the school setting can be more beneficial when coordinated with how interventions are implemented at school. This also requires parental consent and ROI documentation.

Why don't the IEP accommodations seem to be working?

There are so many reasons. The first is that it takes a long time. Medication is the only intervention that really can show an immediate result. Other accommodations rely on your student learning new behaviors and habits to get the benefit from them. As difficult as forming habits is for neurotypical children, those routines are even more difficult for ADHDers to build.

Because I've been very lucky to have had a consistent placement at one school for several years, I did get to see how students learned, progressed, and improved in all areas over the years. One of my favorite memories is of a student who very much had the hyperactive-impulsive flavor of ADHD. One day, toward the end of his fourth grade year, he said to me, "You know what I'm proud of? I haven't punched anybody this year." This was significant because his third grade year was a doozy. (That was also the first year back in school after COVID.)

Case after case, I have had the rewarding experience of seeing kids make huge improvements after years of hard work.

But I've also seen many situations where several different strategies needed to be tried before something started working. Every child is different, and neurodivergent children are even more different from each other than neurotypicals are from each other. Just because one intervention works great for one ADHDer doesn't mean it will automatically work for other ADHDers. And what works for a while might suddenly stop working so well. Kids are changing all the time. Especially when puberty begins and the brain chemistry gets thrown off by new and different levels of hormones.

Another thing to look out for is how the team implements accommodations. A lot of times really great intervention ideas will be proposed in IEP meetings. Amazing ideas. Things that really could help your child. But the implementation gets botched and it becomes just another thing collecting dust (physical or metaphorical) in the classroom.

New tools and techniques need to be taught, which takes time. Unfortunately, time is in short supply. Occupational therapists have the expertise and experience to write up really good sensory routines, but they often have their time split over several schools. If there isn't staff on-site that can help facilitate the sensory routine, and keep to the routine without letting it turn into a loosey-goosey free playtime, it's difficult for the child to get the benefit. Unfortunately, the school-based staff member might not have had a chance to be trained by the OT on how to implement the sensory routine.

There are analogous scenarios for any intervention brought to the IEP meeting by itinerant specialists.

What do I do if the school can't consistently give my student what they need?

If you're the kind of person who can hire a lawyer, you can try getting a lawyer involved. I'm not sure adding the stress of a potential lawsuit inspires the school to have a better approach to your child, but it's a strategy. It can pretty much torpedo some school staff's efforts to form positive connections with your child. It turns out that, no matter how hard we as a culture have tried, we just can't litigate people into being decent to each other.

If you're the kind of parent who can afford a lawyer, you might also be the kind of parent who can afford private school tuition. If you can afford a really good lawyer, you might even be able to get the public school district to pay for it.

Some private schools market themselves as having a more neurodivergent-friendly way of setting up and managing the educational experience. Of course, that's marketing, and results may vary. In some places, there are public charter schools that may also provide a better environment for ADHDers. But there's a wide variety of charter schools with different missions and methodologies.

Schools that focus on hands-on experiential learning can be really great for an ADHDer. However, there is, again, the difference between marketing and implementation. I am personally a big fan of the Montessori Method. (Maria Montessori developed her teaching strategies by working with "defective children" who had been expelled from the state-run schools. So, before there was even a word for neurodivergence, Maria Montessori was figuring out how to successfully educate neurodivergent kids.) But not all Montessori, or Montessori-inspired, schools are the same. Some of them are just using the label to attract customers.

If you're going the private or charter school route, make sure you do some digging on how they actually operate. And take test score data with a grain of salt. The academically rigorous schools with the great test scores tend to shed students like crazy before testing season comes around in the spring. One of my first teaching jobs was at an academically rigorous charter middle and high school. On my first day of inservice, the school's special education teacher basically told me I didn't need to worry too much about the kids with IEPs. "They usually leave the school once the math gets too hard."

There's always the homeschooling option, but, honestly, after working with kids during the COVID shutdowns, I'm not the person to talk to about how to do it. Homeschooling seems a great way to acclimatize kids to the social environment of their own house. Most of my experience with homeschoolers is with students whose parents tried homeschooling them for a year and then realized it wasn't doing anyone any good. Returning to school after a year or two at home is rough. It's also a lot of extra and dysregulating transitions to ask your ADHDer to go through. Life throws enough of those at us as it is.

Really, the best thing to do is act in a way that your child knows you are on their side. Be there for them at the end of a tough day. Don't hang their report card grades over their heads. Be in close contact with the teacher and the school so that they don't feel like they need to call home about every minor behavior problem. Hold your ADHDer accountable when they really screw up, but also, have their back. Listen to their side of the story. Insist the teachers and the principal take into account your child's side of the story. Find positive mentors and activities outside the school. Don't let them feel like how they are at school defines their whole lives.

The school may not be able to change how they do things. Sometimes they just can't. But if you can help your child have a good life at home and outside of the school day, that can make a big difference. It takes some of the pressure off, and your child might actually find it's easier to navigate the school day because of it.

Side Quest:

Litigation

If you are seriously thinking about going the litigation route, I'm surprised you're still reading this book. But if you are, I'm really curious about your angle and how it turns out. There are special education lawyers who take pro bono cases. These cases have led to class actions and major reforms in the public schools. They also tend to add more confusing line items to IEP paperwork. When you go the lawyer route, make sure you consider who it will really benefit and who it will really hurt. In most cases, it benefits the lawyer more than anyone else. The student bears the stigma of becoming a doubly special case that the school staff walks on eggshells around. The parents will never trust the school again. The school district will redirect resources away from directly serving students in order to pay for the legal stuff. It's not the best way to build a positive working relationship.

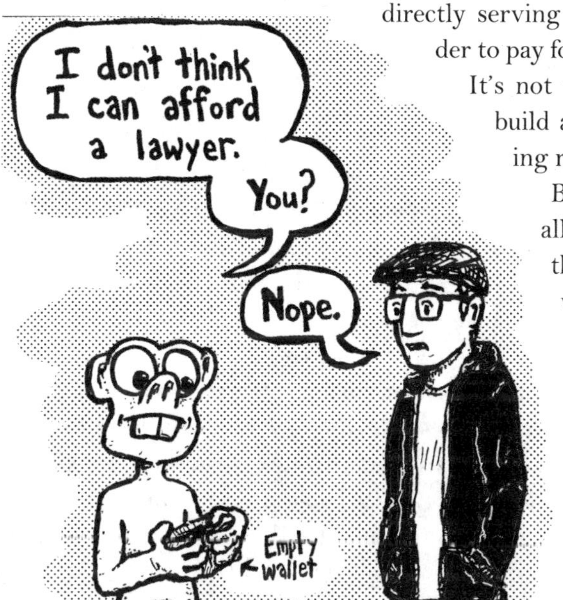
I don't think I can afford a lawyer.
You?
Nope.
Empty wallet

But, if you really need to nail the school to the wall, go for it. It is the American way.

FOR ADHD STUDENTS

The first thing you need to know is that if school feels like it's extra hard for you, that's because it is extra hard for you. I'm just going to validate that feeling for you right now. I can't give you the magic spell to make it stop being hard, but I can help you know what to look for, what to ask for, and what to realistically expect schools to be able to help you with.

First off, find your people. ADHD is as common as left-handedness. There will be plenty of people out there with similar difficulties. Try to get connected with others. You'll be able to trade tricks and tips, and most importantly, you will feel less alone. If your school will let you (and they're supposed to let you), try to form an ADHD peer group or a neurodivergent student peer group.

Second, and especially if you are still in grade school or high school and have an IEP, try to give honest feedback about what the IEP team is providing for you. If you have no idea what's on your IEP, ask. Your parents/guardians are on the IEP team, and they should have access to all the documentation. If your parents/guardians don't understand the documentation (and I wouldn't be surprised, considering how bizarrely written most of the IEPs I've seen are), advocate for yourself at school. Ask the special education teacher to break it down for you so you understand it. If there are parts that absolutely don't make sense to you, make sure they know they don't make sense. Here's a good line to use if they give you pushback, "If I don't understand what this IEP goal means, how can I reach it?"

If you're not on an IEP but have a 504 plan, you have a similar right to question the plan. Luckily, 504 plans are usually simpler and written by school counselors who have a lot better training in talking to students and families in ways that aren't confusing.

If you're in college, you're more on your own across the board. There will be an office of disabled student services of some sort. It will be good to make yourself known there and find out what they have to offer. In college, it is up to the student to be a self-advocate and ask for the accommodations they need.

Unfortunately, new college students have a lot of experience in their previous school setting just having to deal with all the confusing stuff the IEP team does to try and help out. If you're a college freshman, it is likely that you have a poor idea of what help and accommodations you actually need. This is why it's very important to find your people. Hopefully, your campus has a self-advocacy group for ADHDers or neurodivergent students in general that you can join. Every college and university has its own quirks. Talking to other students who have had experience with your school's systems and how to work with them will be invaluable.

Next, and this is the hardest thing for young people to do, know what it is you need when you go to ask for it. Figure out what exactly it is that you need help with. Is it more time on tests and assignments? Is it specific tutoring on course content? Is it a snack break after the first fifty minutes of a ninety-minute lecture class? Is it note-taking help? Try to have a good idea of what will help you when you ask for it. Sometimes what you need is actually something you can provide for yourself way better than whatever the office of disability services can do.

Find classes and activities at school that give you joy. Get involved in things that rev up all your beneficial neurotransmitters. If at all possible, find ways to use your interests and hobbies as fuel for your school work. In my first year of upper division classes at university, I wrote a paper citing my zine collection for a linguistics class. The next year I had an art history professor give me the option of creating a comic that better illustrated the main points of the strange and meandering final paper I was doomed to get a failing grade on. (I think Prof. McElroy must have known I was neurodivergent before I did. I didn't ask for that alternate assignment, but it really saved my ass.)

Finally, don't sweat being perfect. For a long time, I felt like anything less than an A was a failing grade. It's not. Don't be that kind of grade-obsessed perfectionist. Don't burn yourself out on a class that it's impossible for you to get better than a C in. Take the C and move on with your life. Those grades really don't matter that much in the end. Get your diploma or degree and get the hell out of there.

What kind of accommodations should I ask for?

One of the most difficult things is figuring out what kind of help actually helps you. Especially since we have a tendency to measure our capabilities by our highest performing days and not by the days we struggle. But, guess what. Those highest performing days, the ones you are basing your perfect-day expectations on, are the days when all the supports just happened to be lined up for what you needed that day.

Just yesterday I was talking to my college-age daughter because she had a panic attack at a class activity. (She's been calling these episodes panic attacks since long before her ADHD diagnosis, and they seem to be in the vein of the intense social anxiety reactions that feed into rejection crash or RSD.) It was the first one she had had in a while, and it was a lot less intense. We were also able to talk through what happened and analyze the situation.

One thing we identified is that her Adderall had been back-ordered for three weeks. She hadn't been able to take her meds. So, that was something definitely adding context. The next was that this group class activity, striking a set with the drama department, was a big thing she hadn't done before. There were a lot of people, more than just her class, and a lot of power tools making a lot of noise. So it was hard to focus. When she asked teachers for specific instructions on what she could do, what she heard was very vague. Either the teachers weren't specific enough, or her working memory was not able to hold onto the information.

Taking all this into consideration made us realize there were a few accommodations that might actually help. One of them is something she can implement: hearing protection. There are a lot of really great options for noise-reducing ear plugs these days. (Don't waste your time with the disposable foam doodads.) I even got a set of Loops for working cafeteria duty.

Another accommodation was getting written instructions for things going on in noisy environments. If the disabled student service department at her school balks at helping her get written instructions for an assignment, they will be on the receiving end of some very tense phone calls from this dad.

Lastly, the meds shortage. The school really can't get the meds to you faster. But, hopefully, they can be understanding and have some grace while you're dealing with it.

So, sadly, you have to experience some hard days and be able to analyze them in order to figure out what supports you need to help you get through the hardest days.

How do I deal with bullies?

Like Sarah did with Jareth in the movie *Labyrinth.* She told him he had no power over her and the whole Labyrinth crumbled. Easy.

Okay. It really isn't that easy, but *Labyrinth* is a good place to look for inspiration. And there is a core truth to it.

In school, the kids who engage in bullying are experimenting with how to manipulate other people by triggering shame responses. I go into shame a bit in the section where I talk about rejection crash and RSD, so I'll try not to repeat myself too much. But basically,

Side Quest: Find Your People

There are other people with ADHD at your school. Statistically, unless there are only ten people total, students and staff, you are not the only one with ADHD. You've probably already found some other ADHDers. They might not know it. They might not be ready to share it. But they are around.

The biggest thing that saved my life in middle school was when a group of comic book fans found me and took me in as one of their mutants. This was 1988, and the only language we knew to describe living a life that felt out of step with the normals was provided by Chris Claremont's writing in the pages of The Uncanny X-Men. So, there was no talk of diagnoses, but there was a general acceptance that we could be our own weird selves, and it was fine.

Find the people who are like this for you. The people who are really into the weird niche thing you're into. Or, they're into a different weird niche thing, but can totally understand and respect the passion you bring to your hyperfocus activities.

Also, if you can, find some adult ADHDer role models in the staff. They are probably there. Some people with ADHD get drawn into teaching because they want to help out the kids like themselves. Hopefully some of them are comfortable sharing their diagnoses. (You hear me, ADHD educators? Hint. Hint. Our kids need legit role models.) Having an adult around that can relate to having a frenetic symphony in your brain all the time is going to help you see a place for an adult version of you in the world. (Again, ADHDers who have kids in their life or work. Hint, hint. Drop the social mask, and get real with how to be a grown-up in this world.)

Of course, remember those teacher/student boundaries. ADHD adults sometimes need help remembering that you are not their personal offspring child. Hopefully, your elder allies won't need reminders to keep things professional. If they do, it's really not your job to do the reminding. That being said, all of us have to do things that aren't technically our jobs sometimes.

One way to help keep things professional before any problems happen is to make sure your interactions remain visible and happen in common spaces. You could also ask if your ADHD role model/teacher would sponsor an official club or affinity group at school. Having an official club is a great way to make sure things remain legit.

shame is a secondary emotion that comes about as a reaction to how you feel about how you fit with social structures.

I'm not going to go into why bullies do what they do. You don't need to know why someone is being an asshole to know they're being an asshole. It's up to them to figure that out with their therapist or parole board. The less time and energy you spend unpacking a bully's motives, the better.

It's easier to take a look at what they are doing. They are taking actions to humiliate you, to cause you to feel shame about bullshit they are doing to you. If you can remember that they are the ones doing the bullshit, you don't have to take ownership of it. It's their bullshit and it reflects on them, not on you.

The age old advice to ignore bullying behavior is terrible advice for anyone who has a neurological difficulty choosing what they pay attention to. Instead, I urge you to figure out how to respond to them in a way that does not give them any evidence of the shame reaction they are trying to get out of you. They want you to get outraged and mad and to do something embarrassing. Do something confusing instead.

Try to approach the situation with questioning instead of anger. (Not always possible, I understand. But try to fake it.) Saying in a calm, befuddled voice something like, "I'm totally confused by what you're saying. What is it that you need help with?" might just derail them. They didn't get the immediate reaction they were looking for, so they're going to move on.

What about physical bullying?

Get the hell out of there. Report the physical abuse. Get witnesses if you can. This is where having a posse of neurodivergent super friends can come in handy. Bullies will pick on loners. If you've got a posse, they've got too many obstacles to getting to you.

What if the bully is an adult who works at the school?

This shouldn't happen. But it does. And it's often your word against theirs. So, again. Get a posse for witnesses and self-preservation. Hopefully, there will be some sort of mechanism to address the problem with school officials. If not, there's the local news media. Or, maybe it's time to look at the litigation side quest earlier in this book.

Side Quest:

Trade School

If you feel like a four-year university is just not for you, or not for you at this point in your life, that's okay. There are other paths. If I knew at seventeen what I know now, I might have trained as an electrician and had a hell of a good time running wires all over new construction for fifteen years before deciding to become a realtor or something. There are a lot of skilled trades that people with ADHD might find quite appealing: HVAC, plumbing, carpentry, welding! (Do you know how much a good welder can make?)

If you work in the trades, you get to work with your hands. You have visual evidence of what you accomplished at the end of the day. You get to change job sites frequently. Every day has the potential to be a whole new adventure.

If you're good at your trade, you can go into business for yourself. Being your own boss might be the best thing for an ADHDer. Just think about it. If you're thinking college might not be the best place for you, there are lots of other places.

FOR ADHD EMPLOYEES

Unless you are planning for a career in academia, school will end. A very dark joke that comes up in the world of special education is that, as soon as students turn twenty-one, they are all magically cured. We know this isn't true, even if there still is this persistent misconception that only ten-year-old boys have ADHD.

In the workplace, there are plenty of ADHDers clocking in and clocking out. If you don't have ADHD, the odds are pretty good that someone you work with does. If you do have ADHD, the odds are you have trouble sticking at one workplace for more than a couple years. In some cases, a couple months are more than enough to convince an ADHDer it's not the right fit.

Why is it so hard for ADHDers to stay in one job?

First of all, I feel a little called out by that question. But at the same time, I feel seen. For the past twelve years, I have been with the same employer and, nominally, in the same job. However, that job, as a paraeducator for a large urban school district, changes year to year and month to month.

The only reason I've managed to hang on so long is that, no matter what, November is going to look very different from September. And the same can be said for February and May. (April's generally the worst, though.) Also, there are a lot of built-in breaks in the school year.

But, to get back to the question, ADHDers need stimulation and variety. Most of the time, there's a honeymoon period when you start a job, with a heightened level of alertness and focus. This is largely because the new job is new. Everything is novel and stimulating in a way that keeps those neurotransmitters pumping. There's also the sense of urgency around proving yourself early on. Everything about the first week of a new job is really keeping our brains on alert and ready to go.

It's the second week that the troubles begin. (Or maybe the second month. Or the second year. Timeframes will vary per individual.) Once the newness of everything has worn off, the neurotransmitters we know and love, dopamine and norepinephrine, start leaving the party. That's when it starts getting a little harder to make it in on time. The tedium of some parts of the job starts to get to us. We've figured out which people's opinions matter in the workplace and which one's don't. If we're not a big fan of how that shakes out, it adds more resistance and undermines our motivation.

If there's not a sense of novelty or urgency to the job that stimulates us in a meaningful way, we're going to start resenting a lot of what we have to do to earn that paycheck.

So, either we start looking for a new job, we quit out of frustration, or we have some kind of emotional breakdown that leads to disciplinary action or getting fired.

I'm not saying this happens with every place of employment for every ADHDer. It's just a very familiar story. A lot of ADHDers only need to experience this disappointing employment cycle a few times before they figure out how to interrupt it: you've got to be brutally honest with yourself. Figure out your strengths and weaknesses and what you're willing to put up with. Get some good data on how your energy ebbs and flows and what activities affect that ebb and flow. Then use that to figure out what kind of job, or jobs, will work best for you.

Some ADHDers find that a patchwork of part-time jobs and side hustles works better for them than a full-time job. Some identify a job that nobody wants, but is tolerable, and go for it. This kind of job often has fewer applicants competing for it, is possibly mandated by some governmental requirements, and may even be more difficult to be fired or let go from. (This is how I got into being a special education paraeducator.) Some are able to identify a valuable skill that they are very interested in developing, and turn that into a job. Others create their own job, going into business for themselves.

None of this is easy, but you don't necessarily have to do it alone. If you have been able to build some good connections in your community, there will be people you can bounce ideas off of. In addition to these connections, if you live in the United States, you can seek help from your state's vocational rehabilitation services.

What is vocational rehabilitation?

Vocational rehabilitation, or voc rehab, is a governmental service that is required under the Rehabilitation Act of 1973 (the same law that includes the Section 504 that comes into play in public education). As the "For Parents of ADHD Students" section discusses, 504 plans are often implemented for students with ADHD because the threshold for establishing a disability for a 504 is lower than that for an IEP under the IDEA law.

Voc rehab's whole mission is to help people with disabilities find meaningful work. They help with career counseling, skills assessment, job placement, and, if needed, intervening with employers. There are no income limitations on accessing vocational rehabilitation services. You don't have to be unemployed, either. If you feel stalled-out in your career, or that you are in danger of losing your job due to issues relating to disability, voc rehab is there to help you.

Of course, there are always gatekeepers. It can be harder to establish disability with a government entity when you have an invisible disability like ADHD. This is where having a medical diagnosis can help. Also, having a track record of uneven, or stagnant, employment will hopefully make it clear that you are deserving of voc rehab's help.

It's free to apply for vocational rehab and most of the services they provide are either free or at very low cost.

Do I have to disclose to my employer that I have ADHD?

If you want to have access to the antidiscrimination protections in the ADA (Americans with Disabilities Act) or get assistance with your employer through voc rehab, you need to disclose.

But, if you want to manage your career without relying on those resources, you don't have to. Your personal privacy regarding your health, both physical and mental, is your right.

Are there disadvantages to disclosing to my employer?

If your employer is an asshole, yes (in which case, you should be working on your exit strategy anyway).

Several years ago, I was advised by my union local's president not to disclose my invisible disability to HR. Her instinct and experience was that our employer would just use that information to find reasons not related to my disability to try and get rid of me, if that's what they wanted to do. Was this a real possibility? Maybe. At the time, I felt like I didn't need any accommodations beyond what was spelled out in the contract and my job description. It has since become evident to me that the employer in question pulls a lot of dick moves and has no qualms about disregarding contract

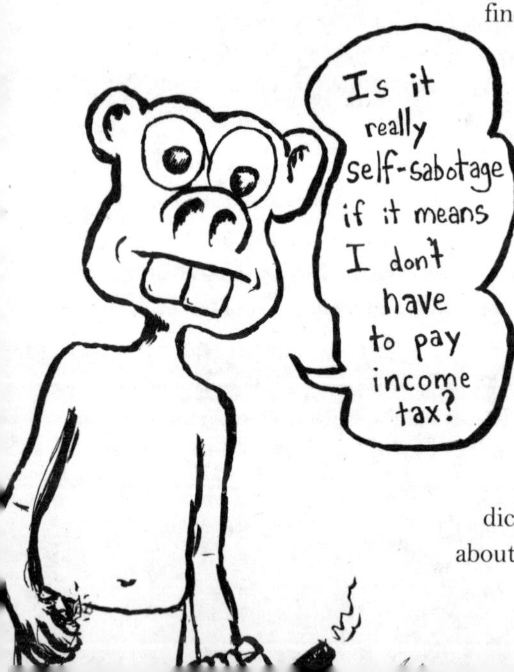
Is it really self-sabotage if it means I don't have to pay income tax?

language when it suits them. But the benefits package is pretty good. Sometimes it's worth it to keep your head down and not rock the boat for a while.

Another reason not to disclose is that you really don't want to explain things to your boss and coworkers. There are a lot of misconceptions out there and you don't want your day job taken over by putting in the extra effort to prove them wrong. If you've got your ADHD traits managed pretty well, the needs of the job line up well with your strengths, and you meet the requirements of your employer, it may not be necessary to disclose.

It can really depend on the workplace culture. Some workplaces actually genuinely embrace the innovative and out-of-the-box thinking that neurodivergent workers bring with them. These workplaces tend to have communication and workflow processes and procedures in place that keep things running smoothly for neurotypical and neurodivergent employees alike. Ironically, these are the employers you probably don't need to disclose to.

Are there advantages to disclosing to my employer?

The biggest advantage to being upfront about your ADHD is that you don't feel like you need to hide something important about yourself. If you don't have to put energy into trying to appear normal, you have more energy for actually getting the job done. In the end, that's what should count.

What if I'm still not comfortable with telling everyone at my workplace?

You really don't have to. You can be true to yourself without oversharing. Most people aren't going to care that much. A lot of workplace issues can be resolved by just focusing on what the physical characteristics of the problem are. Are the lights too bright? Is the A/C too cold? Not cold enough? Is your work station too close to environmental noises (or noisy people)?

And before you even need to bring it up with anyone, you can see if there is anything you can do to address the problem yourself.

Workplaces can vary a lot. Depending on what kind of work it is, you might be able to get the accommodations you need without ever having to mention ADHD. Most employers actually don't want their employees to be miserable. Some of them actually don't understand why the miserable employees stick around. This is especially true in high turnover workplaces like food service or retail.

What are things I can ask for from my employer, even if I don't disclose my ADHD?

There are some basic things that make a workplace easier for everyone, regardless of neurotype. Interestingly enough, not all employers have these in place.

- First off, having a clear job description is great. It doesn't necessarily have to be written down, but it should definitely be discussed. (Really, it should be written down somewhere, for your employer's sake.) The job description will make clear what the job duties are, what your place is in the organizational workflow, who you report to, and who reports to you. This maks it easier to know which tasks and people you should focus on. And, as they say at the end of every episode of the old *G.I. Joe* cartoon, knowing is half the battle.

- Second, ask for flowcharts or checklists for the common tasks involved in your job. This really does put the burden of organization on your boss, but that's the boss's job, right? If they don't want to do this, you've got some choices. You can do the half-assed job your boss obviously expects (and be ready with the explanation of your poor training when the boss wonders why you aren't using your whole ass). You can make your own flowcharts and checklists as you train yourself (and maybe you'll get promoted because you'll end up understanding your job better than the boss does). Or, you can figure out your exit strategy and move on to the next job.

- Third, ask for feedback on how you are handling your workload before problems come up. A lot of times, we like to put up a front of competence when we are actually struggling to keep our heads above water. Don't do that. If there's a certain work-related task, or part of a task, that is constantly giving you trouble, ask for guidance on how to do it more efficiently. And ask early. Employers won't know what specific tasks you need help managing if you don't let them know. It's much better to ask these questions when you're new to a specific task than after you've been faking it for months.

These should all be super basic things helpful to any employee. If an employer can't provide them, there's a good chance that employer might not make it in the long run. Unless they're part of a government entity, or a tech billionaire's pet project. In which case, it never hurts to be working on an exit strategy.

FOR EMPLOYERS OF ADHD FOLX

First off, employers should read the previous section. Especially the part about job descriptions, checklists, and proactive feedback. If you want your employees to be able to do their job well, having these kinds of processes and procedures in place is key. It's not just good for employees with ADHD; it's really important for everyone at a workplace to have this nuts-and-bolts stuff figured out.

At the same time, your documentation needs to be dynamic to fit evolving circumstances. Just make sure that the processes and procedures are updated to reflect the current needs.

What if I don't have any employees with ADHD?

Are you sure you don't?

ADHD is as common as left-handedness. If you've got ten or more employees, chances are really good that there's someone with ADHD on your payroll. They might have good tools in place and don't feel the need to disclose. It's also possible they don't know it yet. A lot of people are getting diagnosed later in adulthood as the stigma lessens around seeking help for mental and behavioral health issues.

If you're going to make assumptions about your employees, it's a safer bet to assume that there are probably some ADHDers and other neurodivergent folx on staff.

How do I accommodate for ADHD as an employer?

I'm not trying to write a business management book here, but

I've been subjected to a lot of management styles. Here are a few techniques to make work better, not just for ADHDers, but for everyone.

- Don't make assumptions and keep the lines of communication open. Every person with ADHD is going to have different struggle areas. Sometimes, they don't know exactly what it is they need an accommodation for. Don't expect a one-time conversation or pep talk to solve any problems. Instead, realize that things may need to get revisited a few times on the path to improvement.
- When possible, give feedback and announce changes outside of the heat of the moment. If it's a hectic moment in the workflow and your employees are fully engaged in what they are doing, they are not going to have available spots in their working memory to take in new information. Wait for a lull to make a quick check-in. Have a regularly scheduled meeting time for nuts-and-bolts announcements. And, by all means, try to keep that nuts-and-bolts meeting to fifteen minutes or less.
- If some of your employees have more questions than a fifteen-minute meeting allows, release the employees who don't have questions. It can be very hard for an ADHDer to receive new information but not be able to start putting it into practice right away. They know themselves and know that if new information is going to stick, they need to do some focused activity to reinforce its transfer from working memory to long-term memory. The sooner the better. Of course, some people do need to verbally rehash and have elaborate or redundant questions answered. You can give those employees that time without holding the rest of the team hostage.

- Have an open door to employee feedback and questions.
- Keep emails to the point. In the days of hand-typed and mimeographed workplace memoranda (the "memos" they talk about in the old shows and movies), it was important to keep them economically short to save paper and labor. Secretaries, as admin assistants were called in those days, had to type out, copy, and distribute all those memos by hand. If your memos were too long, you'd need to hire more admin assistants to get them all out, and that is obviously not very cost effective. These days, the cost of sending an all-staff email is pretty negligible. It is not unheard of for a boss to send out a weekly update email that is several pages long. No one finds this helpful. There is actually a hidden labor cost to this practice because you are potentially losing hours of productivity if your employees are actually reading these things. If you do have that much new information to disseminate, condense it down to bullet points.
- When considering staffing changes, look at the big picture of each employee's performance. Every employee is going to have lulls and surges in their productivity. This is normal. But an ADHDer's lull will look very different from a neurotypical employee's lull. Your neurotypical employee might have a slow start on Monday, a peak on Tuesday, with Wednesday being close behind, a really slow Thursday, and then on Friday, there's a bit of a lift above Thursday in order to get loose ends tied up before the weekend. An ADHDer's cycle may look like a phenomenal Monday, not much visible progress over Tuesday, Wednesday, and Thursday, followed by an explosion of productivity on Friday. It may be that the ADHD employee is actually more productive over the average work week than the

neurotypical employees.

- Have clear boundaries, with built-in guardrails, in place. Keep reinforcing the workplace expectations for interactions between staff and between staff and customers. Model the kind of conduct you want to see from your employees. ADHDers sometimes forget the rules for the social context they are in. They love one-upping boundary-testing behaviors. So, it's really important to have some clear, to-the-point, and easy-to-remember standards. A simple catchphrase like, "Hey, this is a family establishment" might be enough of a guardrail to reign most things back in. However, if you are the kind of boss who likes to dip into petty cash in order to visit your friend "Dusty" on a regular basis, don't be surprised if your employees start skimming money from the cash register.

What if an employee refuses to do an important function of their job because of their ADHD?

First, I'm going to ask if this function is expressly written in the job description and was discussed in the hiring process. If the answer is yes, then your employee might benefit from some job coaching, either from your organization, or from your state's vocational rehab agency.

If the job function in question is something that was within the scope of the job before hiring, it really is the responsibility of the employee to discuss accommodations before signing the contract. While there are laws protecting against hiring discrimination, ADHD is in a legal gray area as far as the Americans with Disabilities Act is concerned. Up-front communication is going to be in everyone's best interest, and if your employee is not good about up-front communication, well, that's not technically an ADA-recognized disability. If they are not the right employee for the job, they're not the right employee for the job. Do your best to work with them, or, perhaps find a different role that suits their strengths and abilities.

If it's a new task that's being added to an existing employee's job description, you've gotta be ready to work with them. Especially if they have an established record of meeting the requirements of the old job description. This is another instance where good communication and specific training can hopefully help you and your employee figure out what works.

If your employee is absolutely unwilling to work with you, there are likely to be multiple areas in which they are falling short. If you have those shortcomings documented along with documentation on how you've tried to address them, you gotta do what you gotta do to keep the business going.

FOR NEUROTYPICAL ALLIES: FRIENDS, PARTNERS, TEACHERS, AND FAMILY MEMBERS

The first thing you need to know is that ADHDers are human beings. You also need to know that the full breadth of the human experience is quite larger than you assume. So, really, it's best not to make a lot of assumptions. Instead, be curious about the ADHDers in your life. Ask them questions and be ready to hear answers that don't jive with your previous assumptions about how people work and do things. Big picture: allow yourself to get to know your ADHDer as a whole person in their own right, and not as a partial person with stuff missing because "they have a disorder."

Does social media cause ADHD?

This is basically the same question as "Do video games cause ADD?" And that's basically the same question as "Does sitting too close to the black-and-white television cause delinquentism?" And we can probably find similar questions all the way back to "Does whipping your head around to track random movements in the distance cause the wolves to get closer to our sheep?"

So, objectively, no. Social media does not cause ADHD. Social media is merely another thread in the tapestry of our lives.

The above question falls back into the assumption that ADHD is caused by environmental factors. On the shorter timeline, when we're taking into account highly stimulating and novel elements being introduced into our environment, like social media or video games or TV, it should not be a huge shock that ADHD brains tend to be very interested in them. But they aren't doing anything to create the traits in the brain that make them appealing. On the longer timeline, however, having one or two people out of every twenty who are especially good at spotting the movements of predators at a distance probably provided an evolutionary advantage. I'm not an evolutionary biologist, but I did self-publish a time travel novel, so I think I know a little something about things like this.

Coming back to the bright, shiny, and highly neurologically rewarding domain of social media, there is an additional answer I can tease out of this question. While social media doesn't cause ADHD, it sure as hell does a great job of spreading awareness. Though social media might not do the best job of fact-checking, it provides more opportunities to see lived-experience perspectives as opposed to the often ableist clinical perspectives of the medical model.

How can I support my loved one with ADHD when they're driving me nuts?

"I want to be supportive, but I don't know how to respond when my friend/relative/partner is constantly late to planned events, complains about problems at work that seem easily avoidable, and doesn't respond to messages/phone calls for days, if ever." This is a recurring theme. The struggles of an ADHDer to manage in the neurotypical-dominated world can come across as aloof disregard for the unspoken rules of common courtesy. It can even seem like they have a habit of being intentionally rude.

And maybe they do. Some people are just rude, and we can't rule that out.

However, if you're honestly asking this question, you've

probably already judged that your ADHD friend/relative/partner is someone worth spending time with. The real issue is, you want to be able to efficiently access the time you spend together, and the ADHD struggles are getting in the way of that.

This is an opportunity for a courageous conversation.

Why does it feel like my ADHD loved one is lying to me?

Why do I keep getting these big open-ended questions that need a lot of unpacking? I wish I could just say, "Because your ADHDer is lying," and avoid the hassle of providing a full, well-thought-out answer.

And this is the first part of the answer.

Sometimes, when we as ADHDers are asked a question, the old DMN gets triggered and we have to go back into the biographical information stored deep in those dreamy parts of the brain and take a little mind wander as every tangent is followed and every stone is sufficiently turned over. Twice. Which is great and thorough and actually very thoughtful, but we're feeling pressure to give an answer in the moment, so that glitchy TPN switch kicks on (while a good part of our mind is still in DMN dreamland) and gives an answer that is expedient. The answer addresses the question.

Would we like to do a certain thing on a certain evening with a certain group of people? The TPN gives the snap answer "yes" while the DMN is still working on remembering the following: *Do we like doing that activity? Is there anything else important going on that day? Do I even enjoy spending time with the people in that group?* The DMN might even start a little predictive roleplay through some scenarios at the event. Then, seeing how those might not work out, the DMN says, "Nope. Better not go to that." Unfortunately, the TPN has already committed you. But, the commitment has already dropped out of working memory before getting transferred to either long-term memory or the personal google calendar, thanks to the DMN taking up all that bandwidth.

So, yes, technically the ADHDer lied when they said they would like to do the thing, but they didn't realize it at the time. And now they have to come up with another lie to explain why they can't go, because telling the truth at this point is embarrassing and kind of shameful.

Which is the next part of the answer. Unfortunately, a lot of ADHDers are carrying around shame over how many times they've dropped the ball on things.

If they are undiagnosed, they really don't know why it keeps happening and feel like failures as human beings, but they know they have to keep trying to be a regular human being, because that's the only kind of human being they've been taught about. They feel a need to cover up their failings, so they create a fabric of low-stakes lies from which they create the mask they use to hide their traits. If they are diagnosed, but still early in the work of figuring out how to work best with their traits, that shame is still there.

Diagnosed or not, shame-based aggression can easily be flipped from inward pointing to outward. When ADHDers are called out on their inconsistencies, they may accuse others of lying. They may be totally convinced that they never confirmed they would go to said event and that the other person is misrepresenting the conversation. This will go on up to and until the body cam evidence is submitted in court. And by that time, the friendship is pretty much ruined.

It's not just with missed appointments. This shame-based defense mechanism can come into play any time an ADHD trait gets negative attention called to it. Lateness, messiness, poor personal hygiene, losing important things, forgetting appointments. These are all things that plague ADHDers. The urge to mask, misdirect, and pretend it's a wild and free bohemian lifestyle choice comes on hard.

Ironically, all of these traits get aggravated when more pressure is applied to an ADHDer. The more the ADHDer, or the neurotypical involved with the ADHDer, focuses on these things, the worse they get, the deeper the shame grows, and the more destructive the masking and overcorrecting behaviors become.

How do I help my ADHDer get over the shame?

Lots of hugs are a good start.

Seriously, the oxytocin boost from a good hug does wonders for the brain. And it helps reinforce those necessary feelings of connection. If you are on a consensual hugging basis with your ADHDer, hugs are great.

Short of hugs, remember that the shame an ADHDer is prone to comes from a lifetime of events. Shame is an emotional reaction an individual has when they feel like they are not meeting the expectations of their social landscape. It functions by making the shamee want to remove themselves from society. A lot of neurotypicals do this in a quiet, internal way. They shove their sense of self into a corner in their minds and get to business doing whatever it is their boss/teacher/community/grandma wants them to do, then let their sense of self come back later when the moment has passed. Of course, western European cultures do a crap job of teaching and modeling how to do this efficiently. And ADHDers already have trouble doing things efficiently, especially when it involves intangible things like emotions.

So, if a physical hug is off the table, you can be validating and reassuring. Don't discount the depth of their feelings. The dodgy mix of neurotransmitters actually does make those feelings pretty difficult to manage, and telling an ADHDer to shake it off or to buck up buttercup is not going to help them.

However, letting them know they are safe to feel that shame in your presence can help them get past it faster. Help them remember where they are now, that a lot of shame is a built-up reaction to past situations, and that the present is a different situation.

If you are available to do it, let them know you can help problem-solve the current issue once those past-based shame feelings have run their course.

What if my ADHDer starts hyperfocusing on an expensive hobby?

This happens. There is loads of anecdotal evidence on Instagram and TikTok of ADHDers splurging on all the gear for a new passion project, only for it to end up collecting dust in the closet, garage, or storage unit before the credit card statement arrives.

But does it actually happen as often as your anxiety about it makes you feel? Does your ADHDer actually go and pull the trigger on supplies purchases in the middle of a hyperfocus fugue? Or do you catch them comparison shopping and make a discouraging comment which starts a whole argument about how you can't afford that right now?

Your answers to these questions may vary. There may be an established pattern that shows your ADHDer really could use some better guardrails. But setting up those guardrails shouldn't happen during a conversation about a new hyperfocus topic. You can try, but it's very likely to start a fight or an RSD response, neither of which will lead to anything productive.

Rather than trying to immediately shut it down, try to have a nonjudgmental conversation about the new project or hobby. Let yourself be genuinely curious in this conversation. Ask questions along the lines of "How does it work?" rather than "Why would you want to do that?"

When your ADHDer is newly excited about something, let them be excited. Of course, the credit card statement already doesn't look good. But that doesn't mean you need to kill the buzz right away. Just encourage some more imagining about it before pulling the credit card out.

Let the excitement run its course for a while. Let your ADHDer do some deep-dive research. Let them jazz up their norepinephrine on some instructional YouTube videos. Hit the library. Look to see if an introductory class is offered nearby.

See if the excitement builds in momentum in response to the potential reality of doing the things. Or does the enthusiasm fizzle on its own?

A lot of times, the ADHDer really just wants to get all the information on a new, exciting idea before they decide if it fits into their reality. There is a danger that they will spend money before they've reached the commitment threshold. But this danger is greater if they feel like there is a time limit on how long they're allowed to think about it. Instead of saying "no" and hitting them with a rejection crash/RSD trigger, help them find low-cost ways to get the information they need. If you make them feel like it's safe to ruminate for longer, the better they will feel about the whole thing when they make their decision.

How do I set up guardrails with my ADHDer?

Be clear about your expectations. Be clear about what you can deal with. And be willing to have conversations about where you can meet in the middle on some of the issues.

As Warehouse Steve would always say back in my days working at Arizona's largest used entertainment store, "Sometimes you gotta pick which hill you want to die on." What can you live with, and what do you really feel like fighting for? Are your expectations worth giving an ultimatum? Maybe they are. Or maybe you can choose to reframe things.

If you really can't deal with consistently waiting a half hour past the expected time you were supposed to meet your friend at the restaurant, you can stop meeting them at restaurants. Or you can plan to show up a half hour late yourself. If you can't stand a messy house, let your ADHDer have a defined zone where they can have their piles. If they tend to check out in the middle of conversations, you can pick less boring things to talk about.

I joke, but also, we ADHDers do need reminders. More important than what the reminders are about, give those reminders with compassion and respect. Your ADHDer is not trying to constantly disappoint you. They are very likely already beating themselves up over how they keep falling short on some of these things. Have an honest conversation with them and try to work out some parameters for making sure both of your needs are getting met.

I, myself, am very frequently about seven minutes behind schedule. I feel guilty about it. I've had employers talk to me about it. I have no idea how it happens. Lately, I have the brilliant excuse of having a baby in the house. People give you a pass on a lot of things when you have a cute baby in tow. But I was seven minutes late to things before this little girl was here, and I'll probably be seven minutes late after she leaves for college. If someone makes it clear to me they really need me to be on time, I try a little harder. I tell myself to leave the house ten minutes earlier than I think I need to. Most of the time it works. What works better is leaving the house a half hour before I think I need to, but who has that kind of time?

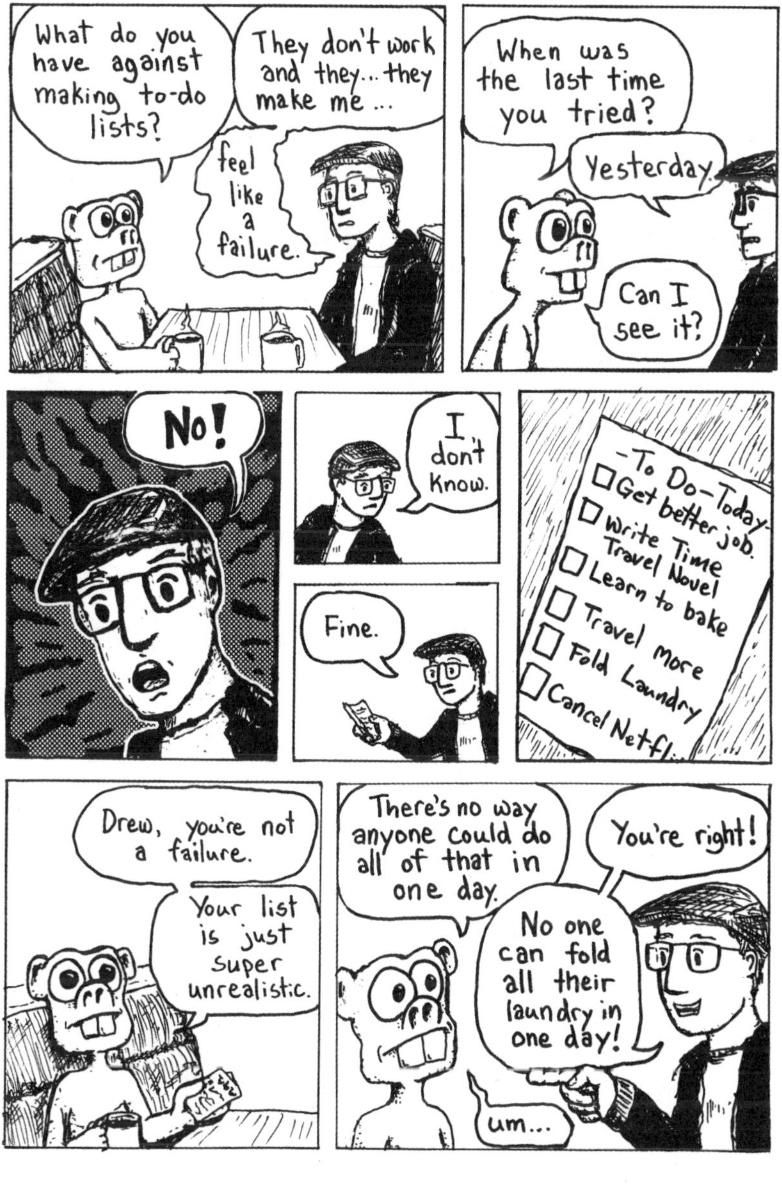
What do you have against making to-do lists?
They don't work and they... they make me ...
feel like a failure.
When was the last time you tried?
Yesterday.
Can I see it?
No!
I, don't know.
Fine.
-To Do-Today-
Get better job.
Write Time Travel Novel
Learn to bake
Travel more
Fold Laundry
Cancel Netfl...
Drew, you're not a failure.
Your list is just super unrealistic.
There's no way anyone could do all of that in one day.
You're right!
No one can fold all their laundry in one day!
um...

CONCLUSION

When I started my first outline of this book, I really wanted to borrow the section heading from Joe Biel and Faith Harper's *The Autism FAQ* (2022): "How do we conclude this book?" Just seeing that section title when I first flipped through the book made me laugh. It was the perfectly autistic way to announce the end of the book.

But this isn't an autism book. It's an ADHD one, and it deserves its own ADHD ending.

So here we go. All joking aside, writing this book has also been an exercise in doing a deep dive and learning a lot of tools that helped me manage my life better.

Do I practice every strategy I've mentioned in this book? Honestly, I do some of them when I remember them. And I try to remember the ones that I notice work really well for me. Here are the top three that really surprised me with how effective they were:

- Taking a moment early in the day to write out a loose plan of what I want to get done. Yeah. A to-do list. For real. I'm still a little chagrined that the to-do list thing works as well as it does. But it really shows on the days when I don't write out a plan (and check back in on it over the course of the day).
- Daily balance exercises. Mind blown. I don't have to go to the gym every day to get the emotional regulation benefits from exercise. I can do a simple beginners Tai Chi routine in my own home. In my jammies. It has really helped me be focused and present in the face of the daily news outrage onslaught.

- The meds have helped me with sensory overwhelm. I didn't expect that. I also never expect when a huge, meltdown-triggering sensory overload is going to happen. But, it would regularly build up during family visits. Since I started taking the meds, I haven't flipped out at my mom for talking to me while I'm trying to unload the dishwasher. Which is good. Because my mom doesn't deserve that. She's a good mom.

My hope, dear reader, is that you have also discovered (or rediscovered) some strategies in this book that work well for you. Try to remember them. If remembering a whole book of stuff is not your style, feel free to randomly flip through it to find that little gem that will jump off the page and get you through the day. Or, if you'd rather have something more portable, shuffle-able, and stimmy satisfying, check out the *ADHD Coping Skills Deck* that I put together with the help of Dr. Faith.

I also hope you've gotten a better picture of how to navigate the confusing, and conflicting, interplay of government, health, and education systems when it comes to ADHD (and a lot of other invisible disabilities). This is a murky, constantly shifting landscape that, hopefully, will make more sense in the future.

If you feel like you're struggling too hard with these systems, or just life, you don't have to struggle alone. There are plenty of in-person and online support groups. Organizations like CHADD (Children and Adults with Attention-Deficit/Hyperactivity Disorder) have chapters and support groups in many places. Or just ask around. Chances are, you already know someone else with ADHD and they would love to talk with you at length.

For real. As soon as I started telling people I was writing this book, a huge chunk of my friend group suddenly decided it was a good time to tell me that they have ADHD. Long story short, you're really not alone.

And, one last thing, sticker charts are awesome!

My sticker chart helped me write an entire first draft fueled by curiosity, enthusiasm, and a desire to put one more sticker on the wall. Seriously, I ADHD-hacked my way all through this project. The fact that this book even exists is strong anecdotal evidence that it works! And I am so glad that it works.

ACKNOWLEDGMENTS

There's a raft of usual suspects who deserve a mention. Lots of people helped me chug through this process, whether they knew it or not.

First, I need to thank my older daughter, Star, who went on her ADHD diagnosis journey the hard way. Our frequent conversations have enriched the text of this book through and through. And thanks to my younger daughter, CJ (not her real name), for finally joining our family and giving me a really good reason to take some time off from my day job. To Kathryn for always being ready to really listen and understand me. To my brother, Marcus, for pointing out to me that my "DHD is Advanced." And to our parents for putting up with us. Then there's my cousin, David, who had a rougher diagnosis journey than most. He's been great for bouncing ideas off of.

Thanks to Ben Cheknis for letting me plug my projects on the *Two Vague Podcast*, even if I do space out sometimes when he's talking about video games. To Angela Morris, for being my work bestie and taking on the crusade of trying to do what's right for all the neurodivergent kiddos in the school. Thanks to Greta West and Cheryl Moren for being fabulous parent advocates, and to their kids for being awesome. ZuZu Cartoons for chatting about adult ADHD life, and validating my intuition at so many turns. Blair, formerly of Rudy's Barbershop, for suggesting I try a sticker chart to track my progress. And, of course, Faith Harper for answering my questions, pointing out stuff I missed, posting sick memes, sending cool stickers, and other bullshittery.

Thanks to Joe Biel at Microcosm for finding just the right prompt to get me to finally write a book. To Elly Blue for answering my questions about how to have an actually neurodivergent-friendly workplace and how to format my manuscript, and for encouraging me to be patient and not mess with anything until my editor had a pass at it. Thanks to Ivy Zeller for being that editor and helping me get this book across the finish line.

And thanks to Bernie just for being Bernie and for making randos at the dog park think I'm his second dad.

REFERENCES

Barkley, Russell. "The Other Attention Disorder: Cognitive Disengagement Syndrome (CDS) - Part I: History & Symptoms." YouTube, July 9, 2023. https://www.youtube.com/watch?v=tQDuF-MKBDI.

Barkley, Russell. "Reduced Life Expectancy in ADHD." CARLAT PUBLISHING RSS, October 11, 2024. https://www.thecarlatreport.com/articles/3096-reduced-life-expectancy-in-adhd.

Barry, Megan K. "What It's Like Having Adult ADHD." What It's Like Having Adult ADHD – Crucial Comix, September 16, 2024. https://www.crucialcomix.com/comic/what-its-like-being-an-adult-with-adhd/.

Becker, Stephen P. "Cognitive Disengagement Syndrome: A Construct at the Crossroads." APA Psychnet, 2025. https://psycnet.apa.org/fulltext/2025-98340-001.html.

Biel, Joe, and Faith G. Harper. *The Autism FAQ: Everything You Wanted to Know about Diagnosis & Autistic Life.* Portland, OR: Microcosm Publishing, 2022.

Broadbent, Elizabeth. "Shame: The Devil on My Shoulder." ADDitude, November 17, 2022. https://www.additudemag.com/rejection-sensitive-dysphoria-adhd-anxiety-depression/.

CDC. "Data and Statistics on ADHD." Centers for Disease Control and Prevention, May 16, 2024. https://www.cdc.gov/adhd/data/index.html.

Cirillo, Francesco. "What Can I Expect from Joining the You & Me Pomodoro® Mentoring Program, and How Is It Different from

Other Time Management Courses?" Francesco Cirillo, 2023. https://www.francescocirillo.com/about-francesco-cirillo.php.

Dodson, William. "How ADHD IGNITES RSD: Meaning & Medication Solutions." ADDitude, July 10, 2024. https://www.additudemag.com/rejection-sensitive-dysphoria-and-adhd/.

Dodson, William. "Free Resource: Understanding Rejection Sensitive Dysphoria." ADDitude, February 16, 2024. https://www.additudemag.com/download/rejection-sensitive-dysphoria-treatment-symptoms/.

Editors, ADDitude. "Does ADHD Need a New Name?" ADDitude, September 19, 2023. https://www.additudemag.com/other-names-for-adhd-add/.

Gendron, Alice. *The Mini ADHD Coach: Tools and Support to Make Life Easier: A Visual Guide.* San Francisco, CA: Chronicle Prism, 2023.

Hallowell, Edward M., and John J. Ratey. *ADHD 2.0: New Science and Essential Strategies for Thriving with Distraction—From Childhood through Adulthood.* New York: Ballantine Books, 2022.

Hallowell, Edward, and John Ratey. "ADHD Needs a Better Name. We Have One." ADDitude, September 30, 2024. https://www.additudemag.com/attention-deficit-disorder-vast/.

Hallowell, Edward M., and John J. Ratey. *Driven to Distraction: Recognizing and Coping with Attention Deficit Disorder from Childhood through Adulthood.* New York: Anchor Books, 2011.

Hallowell, Edward, and John Ratey. "'The Flip Side of Rejection Sensitive Dysphoria: How to Tap into ADHD Energy and Motivation' [Video Replay & Podcast 278]." ADDitude, October 17, 2022. https://www.additudemag.com/webinar/recognition-responsive-euphoria-adhd-podcast-278/.

Harper, Faith G. *Unfuck Your Shame: Using Science to Accept our Feelings, Resolve Guilt, and Connect with Ourselves.* Portland, OR:

Microcosm Publishing, 2024.

Harper, Sammuel E., and Faith G. Harper. *How to Not Be a Dick.* Portland, OR: Microcosm.Pub, 2018.

Keats, Ryan. *The Land before Time Management: Adhdinos.* New York: Union Square & Co. (ADS), 2024.

Larson, Chris. "Done Global Arrests Will Cast a Long Shadow on Behavioral Health." Behavioral Health Business, June 27, 2024. https://bhbusiness.com/2024/06/27/done-global-arrests-will-cast-a-long-shadow-on-behavioral-health/.

Marisa. "7 Myths about Vocational Rehabilitation." YouTube - Disabled In Nature, October 6, 2024. https://youtu.be/7OKPr3JqVk4?si=x2WyOISzDkboEuew.

McCabe, Jessica. *How To ADHD: An Insider's Guide to Working with Your Brain (Not Against It).* New York: Rodale, 2024.

Milgrom, Anne. "Statement from DEA Administrator Anne Milgram on Done Global Inc." DEA, June 14, 2024. https://www.dea.gov/documents/2024/2024-06/2024-06-14/statement-dea-administrator-anne-milgram-done-global-inc.

Pink, Richard, and Roxanne Emery. *Dirty Laundry: Why Adults with ADHD Are So Ashamed and What We Can Do to Help.* Emeryville, CA: Ten Speed Press, 2023.

Walker, Beth. *The Girls' Guide to ADHD: Don't Lose This Book!* Princeton, NJ: Recording for the Blind & Dyslexic, 2006.

Welsner, Lindsay. "Is Rejection Sensitive Disorder Real or Really in Your Head?" Psychology Today, September 25, 2024. https://www.psychologytoday.com/us/blog/the-venn-diagram-life/202409/is-rejection-sensitive-disorder-real-or-really-in-your-head.

ZuZu Cartoons. Accessed October 18, 2024. https://zuzucartoons.com/.

CREATE THE WORLD YOU WANT TO SEE AT MICROCOSM.PU

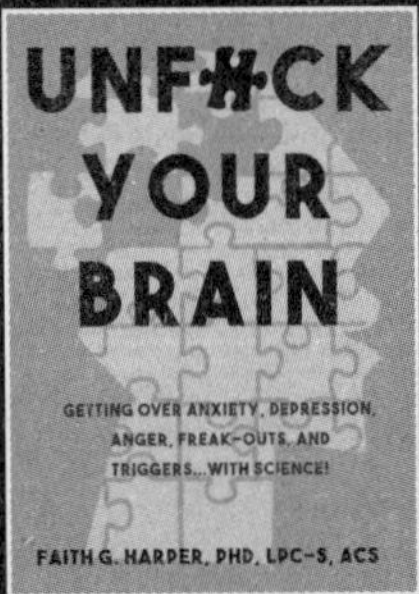

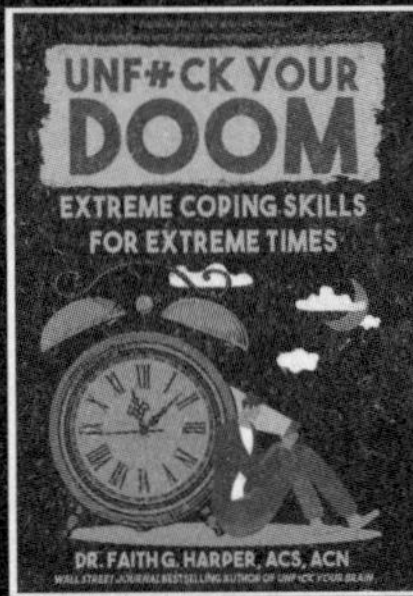

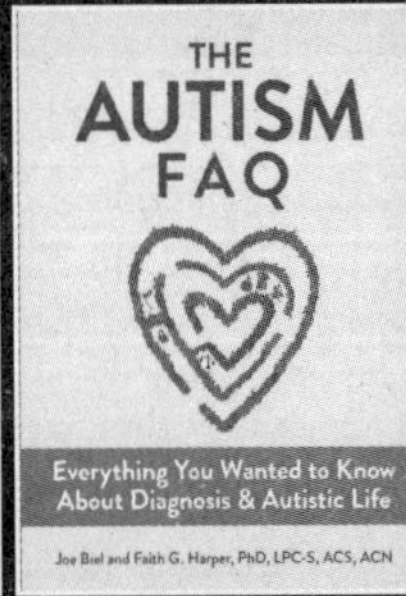

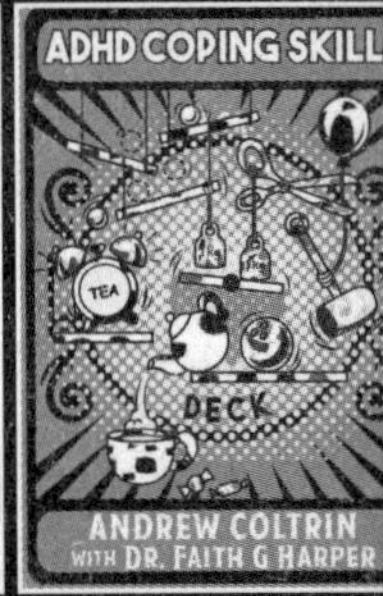

SUBSCRIBE!

For as little as $15/month, you can support a small, independent publisher and get every book that we publish—delivered to your doorstep!

www.Microcosm.Pub/BFF

MORE BEST SELF-HELP FROM WWW.MICROCOSM.PUB

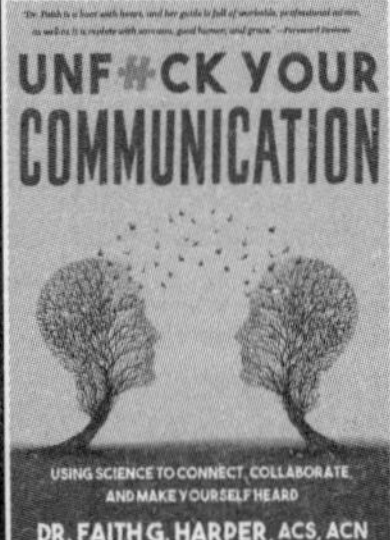

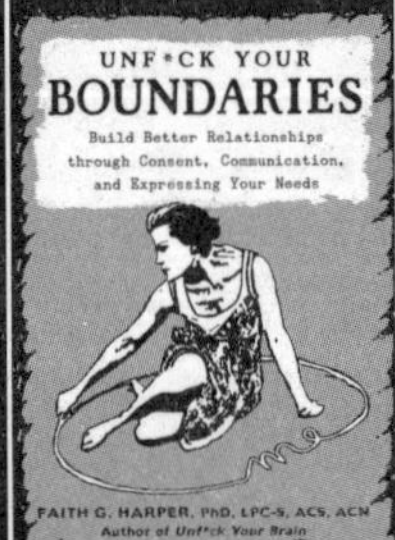

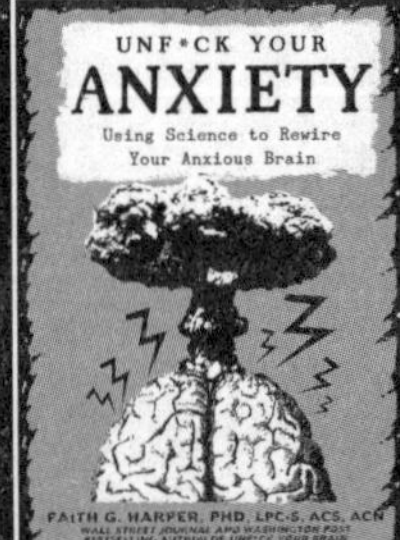

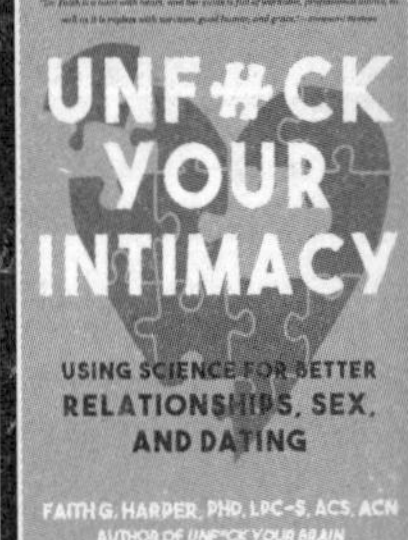